To all the creatures of the sea

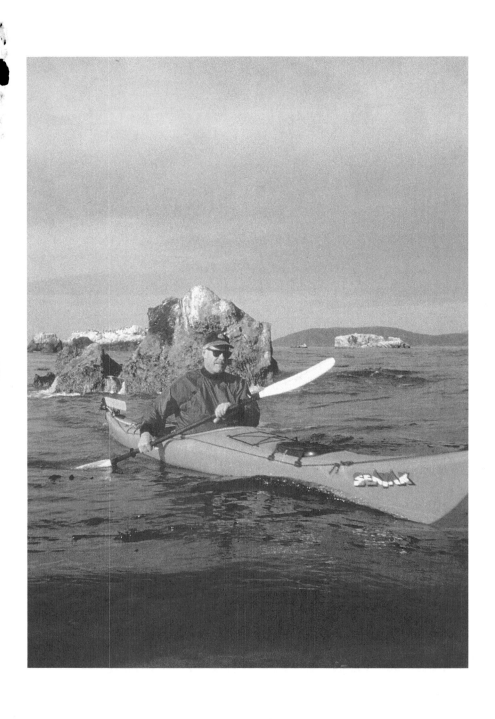

Adventure Kayaking

Trips from Big Sur to San Diego

Includes the Channel Islands

Robert Mohle

WILDERNESS PRESS ... *on the trail since 1967*

Adventure Kayaking: Trips from Big Sur to San Diego

1st EDITION 1998
  2nd printing 2002
  3rd printing 2006
  4th printing 2008

Front cover photo copyright © 1998 by Bill Crane Imagemakers Photography
Back cover photo copyright © 1998 by Bret Royle
Interior photos, except where noted, by Robert Mohle
Maps: Ben Pease
Cover design: Larry B. Van Dyke
Book design: Margaret Copeland/Terragraphics

Library of Congress Card Number 98-17885
ISBN 978-0-89997-224-4

Manufactured in the United States of America
Distributed by Publishers Group West

Published by: **Wilderness Press**
              1345 8th Street
              Berkeley, CA 94710
              (800) 443-7227; FAX (510) 558-1696
              info@wildernesspress.com
              www.wildernesspress.com

Visit our website for a complete listing of our books and for ordering information.

Cover photos: Shell Beach, San Luis Obispo County (Tour SL9) *(front and back)*

Library of Congress Cataloging-in-Publication Data
Mohle, Robert, 1949–
    Adventure kayaking : trips from Big Sur to San Diego / Robert Mohle. -- Ist ed.
        p.   cm.
    Includes bibliographical references (p.) and index.
    ISBN 0-89997-224-1 (alk. paper)
    1. Kayaking--California--Guidebooks. 2. California--Guidebooks.
    I. Title
    GV776.C2M54 1998
    917.9404'53--dc21   98-17885
                                                                 CIP

Table of Contents

Introduction

It was one of those rare spring days. Clear skies and a calm sea stretched as far as the eye could see. The hills were velvety green and the air was cool and crisp. We meandered through the thick beds of kelp, stopping occasionally to peer through the transparent water. The rays of the early morning sun illuminated the shallow reef beneath us that was alive with plants and animals of all shapes, sizes, and colors. A curious harbor seal surfaced nearby, staring at us with his large, round eyes, then quietly disappeared beneath the thick canopy of kelp. Soon we reached a rocky headland. The waves had eroded a small cave in the rock, which we entered. Inside the cave the air was cool and moist. The gurgling water echoed off the damp walls of the chamber, which were covered with a lavender lichen that seemed to glow in the dim light. A second opening to the cave appeared ahead which we paddled through and found ourselves in a small protected cove with a white sand beach.

The sun was higher now, and the air warm and still. A group of brown pelicans silently glided past, their wing tips barely skimming the smooth, glassy water. We stopped for a while and closed our eyes to capture the moment. All of a sudden we heard a loud swooshing sound as two gray whales passed us, leaving cloud of spray as they disappeared beneath the surface of the water. Moments later they reappeared only a few feet from where we sat, breathless. A young calf, perhaps 20 feet long, raised its head from the water to get a closer look at us while its mother patiently waited. We sat motionless while they circled us, then slowly continued on their way.

By the time we reached the landing site, the sun was low in the sky. We were tired but felt relaxed as we loaded our boats onto the car. A man and his son were parked next to us. The man surveyed our kayaks as we continued to load our gear. He asked us what we liked the most about kayaking. After our exciting adventure neither of us was quite sure where to start. Was it the peacefulness, or the freedom, or the close interaction with nature? We looked at each other, and after a few moments of deep reflection my friend responded "Being in the moment. That's what I like most about kayaking." The man hesitated, apparently thinking it over, then said, "Being in the moment? I like that. If that's what kayaking is about, I think I'd like to try it."

This book is about being in the moment; about listening to the wind, watching the waves, and feeling the movement of the sea. On the water there are no roads or fences or signs. You don't need a license and you don't need any gas. You are free, like the birds soaring above and the fish swimming below. You can ride the waves or explore the caves. You can follow the shoreline or paddle far to sea. The choices are endless as you are one with the environment.

The sport of kayaking has opened a whole new world for me: new friendships, new perspectives, good health, and an awareness of my surroundings that I have been able to incorporate into other aspects of my life. I hope this guidebook will be helpful to others, creating opportunities for adventures and an appreciation of the wonders of nature that surround us.

I used to sit on the bluff and watch the sun set over the ocean. Now, in my kayak, I'm part of the sunset. Happy paddling.

Using this Guidebook

Chapter 1 describes the essential components of a successful kayak adventure. Chapters 2-10 contain 52 guided kayak tours throughout the Southern California area. At the end of the book, the Appendix lists kayak retailers and selected references.

The kayak tours are grouped into chapters by county, beginning with Monterey County in the north and proceeding to San Diego County in the south. Also included are a chapter on the Channel Islands and a chapter on kayaking some of the lakes and rivers of southern and central California. At the beginning of each chapter is a regional map showing the locations of the tours and the major roadways in the area. The regional map also includes a listing of the tours in the chapter, the length of each, and the skill level required for each tour.

The tours are presented in a standardized format for simplicity and easy reference. Each tour is given a number and title. Within each chapter, tours are numbered from north to south. The prefix to the number identifies the county (except for Channel Islands tours with the prefix CI and lake and river tours with the prefix LR). A guide map, showing the route, launch and landing sites, and points of interest along the route, accompanies each tour. Following is an example of the format and the kind of the information provided for each tour:

Summary: The summary provides a brief description of the tour.

Skill level: The skill level defines the level of competence required for the tour: beginner, intermediate and advanced. It should be noted that the ocean is constantly changing and conditions that are suitable for a beginner on one day can be challenging or even life-threatening on another. The paddler must understand his or her limitations and use good judgment whenever entering the water.

A beginner-level tour is a relatively easy paddle with minimum hazards under normal conditions. Paddlers should have completed a basic coastal kayaking course equivalent to *The Fundamentals of Coastal Kayaking* course taught by the American Canoe Association. The training should include: how to equip and dress for various conditions; landing and launching through the surf; self rescue; basic paddle strokes and maneuvering; safety, basic navigation, and understanding ocean conditions. Beginner paddlers should have some open-ocean paddling (not the first time) experience and should be in relatively good physical condition.

An intermediate-level tour is a moderately difficult paddle, with open-ocean conditions of limited duration to be expected. An intermediate-level paddler should have all the skills and training of a beginner paddler as well as the ability to conduct a self-rescue (or to rescue another) in windy conditions with open-ocean swells and waves. The paddler should be comfortable launching and landing through the surf on rocky or sandy shores. The intermediate paddler should be in good physical condition and be able to paddle for a moderate period of time against a headwind and opposing currents.

An advanced-level tour is a difficult to very difficult tour, with open ocean conditions of extended duration to be expected. An advanced paddler should have all the skills and training of an intermediate paddler and also be very experienced in reading ocean conditions, planning a trip, and navigating. The advanced paddler should be in very good physical condition and be able to paddle for an extended period of time against a headwind and opposing currents.

Trip length and type: The trip length and type includes the distance in statute (land) miles, the trip type (round-trip or one-way), the setting (open-ocean, bay, or harbor) and the amount of time necessary to complete the tour assuming an average traveling speed of three miles per hour with some time allotted for sightseeing and rest breaks. Your actual time may vary, depending on weather, paddling ability, and float plan.

How to get there: Street directions from the nearest major highway are provided to the launch site. Directions are also provided to the landing site if the trip is one-way and a car shuttle or pick-up are necessary. Information about the availability of parking, restrooms, picnic facilities, lifeguard services, food stores, telephones, and fees is included.

Camping: Nearby state and private campgrounds are identified and a telephone number for reservations is provided (if available).

Chart/map: The National Oceanographic and Atmospheric Administration (NOAA) nautical chart number(s) and the United States Geological Survey (USGS) 7.5 Minute Series quadrangle name(s) for the area included in the tour are both identified.

Hazards: The primary hazards that may be encountered are identified and described. The listed hazards are not necessarily all-inclusive, nor will the listed hazards necessarily be encountered. The list of hazards is intended to assist the reader in preparing for the trip and understanding it's environment. It is the responsibility of the paddler to learn to read and to anticipate ocean conditions, to be fully prepared, and to decide whether the potential hazards of the tour are within his or her capability and comfort level.

Alternate tour: In case conditions are unfavorable, the location of a nearby alternate tour is provided.

Public access: During any kayak tour the need may arise to land on the beach for a rest break, exploration of the shoreline, or an emergency. This section identifies possible landing sites along the route with available public access. Transportation of a kayak to/or from the beach is not practical at most en-route landing sites. Because wave conditions and accessibility can change, it is suggested that whenever possible, proposed landing sites be observed prior to embarking on a tour.

Approximately 42 percent of California's shoreline is publicly owned and accessible. The remaining 58 percent is privately owned or held by a government agency that does not allow public access. All tidal and submerged land seaward of "mean high tide" is public. Although determining the location of "mean high tide" can be difficult, a general rule to follow is that the public has the right to walk on the wet beach.

Kayak surfing: The locations where good waves for kayak surfing can be found are identified along the route.

Launching: A description of the launch site is provided to help you prepare for a safe and successful launch.

Tour description: The tour description guides the reader through the route and identifies points of interest including local history features, marine wildlife, geology, and various shoreline features. Potential hazards along the route are also identified and discussed in the context of the surroundings.

Landing: A description of the landing site is provided to help you prepare for a safe and successful landing.

What to do afterward: Nearby places to see and visit are identified.

For more information: The names and telephone numbers of local groups and agencies are provided.

List of Tours

Monterey County Tours	Skill Level	Length
MO1: Mill Creek to Lopez Point	Intermediate	10.5 miles
MO2: Sand Dollar Beach to Jade Cove	Advanced	2.2 miles

San Luis Obispo County Tours	Skill Level	Length
SL1: Piedras Blancas Point to San Simeon Cove	Intermediate	8.5 miles
SL2: San Simeon Cove	Beginner	1.5 miles
SL3: San Simeon Cove to Leffingwell Landing	Advanced	6.0 miles
SL4: Shammel Park to Cayucos Pier	Advanced	17.2 miles
SL5: Morro Bay Harbor and Estuary	Beginner	11.3 miles
SL6: Montana de Oro	Advanced	4.1 miles
SL7: Spooner's Cove to Olde Port Beach	Advanced	17.0 miles
SL8: Olde Port Beach to Pirate's Cove	Beginner	9.3 miles
SL9: Shell Beach	Beginner	4.4 miles

Santa Barbara County Tours	Skill Level	Length
SB1: Point Sal Beach to Mussel Point	Advanced	8.5 miles
SB2: Jalama Beach Park to Gaviota Beach St. Park	Advanced	20.0 miles
SB3: Refugio State Beach to El Capitan St. Beach	Beginner	6.0 miles
SB4: El Capitan State Beach to Goleta Beach County Park	Advanced	13.8 miles
SB5: Goleta Beach to Arroyo Burro Beach County Park	Intermediate	5.4 miles
SB6: Arroyo Burro Beach County Park to Santa Barbara Harbor	Beginner	4.6 miles
SB7: Santa Barbara Harbor to Carpinteria Beach	Intermediate	11.0 miles

The Channel Islands Tours	Skill Level	Length
CI1: Anacapa: Landing Cove to West End	Advanced	11.2 miles
CI2: Anacapa: Landing Cove to Pinniped Point	Beginner	2.2 miles
CI3: Santa Cruz: Scorpion Bay to Cavern Point	Beginner	3.5 miles
CI4: Santa Cruz: Cueva Valdez to Arch Rock	Intermediate	4.7 miles
CI5: Santa Rosa: Ford Point to Johnson's Lee	Intermediate	4.0 miles
CI6: Santa Barbara: Circumnavigation	Intermediate	6.0 miles
CI7: Santa Catalina: Isthmus Cove to Catalina Harbor	Advanced	17.5 miles
CI8: Santa Catalina: Isthmus Cove to Blue Cavern Point	Beginner	4.8 miles
CI9: Santa Catalina: Catalina Harbor to Little Harbor	Advanced	9.7 miles

Ventura County Tour	Skill Level	Length
VN1: Point Mugu to Leo Carillo State Beach	Intermediate	8.2 miles

Los Angeles County Tours	Skill Level	Length
LA1: Leo Carillo State Beach to Westward Beach	Intermediate	8.5 miles
LA2: Westward Beach to Malibu Pier	Intermediate	9.7 miles
LA3: Marina del Rey	Beginner	4.7 miles
LA4: Malaga Cove to Abalone Cove	Advanced	8.3 miles
LA5: Abalone Cove to Royal Palms State Beach	Intermediate	4.5 miles
LA6: Royal Palms State Beach to Cabrillo Beach	Beginner	2.7 miles
LA7: Port of Los Angeles	Intermediate	6.5 miles
LA8: Alamitos Bay	Beginner	5.5 miles

Orange County Tours	Skill Level	Length
OR1: Upper Newport Bay	Beginner	5.8 miles
OR2: Newport Harbor	Beginner	6.7 miles
OR3: Newport Harbor to Reef Point	Intermediate	4.5 miles
OR4: Reef Point to Aliso County Beach	Intermediate	6.5 miles
OR5: Aliso County Beach to Doheny State Beach	Advanced	6.8 miles

San Diego County Tours	Skill Level	Length
SD1: La Jolla Shores to Mission Bay	Intermediate	11.0 miles
SD2: Mission Bay	Beginner	8.2 miles
SD3: Dana Landing to Mission Bay Entrance	Beginner	3.5 miles
SD4: San Diego Bay	Advanced	15.6 miles

Lakes and Rivers Tours	Skill Level	Length
LR1: Lake Nacimiento, San Luis Obispo County	Intermediate	16.5 miles
LR2: Santa Margarita Lake, San Luis Obispo County	Beginner	12.4 miles
LR3: Lopez Lake, San Luis Obisbo County	Beginner	14.3 miles
LR4: Mammoth Pool Reservoir, Fresno/ Madera Counties	Beginner	12.5 miles
LR5: Lake Hodges, San Diego County	Beginner	14.0 miles
LR6: Lake Morena, San Diego County	Beginner	8.5 miles
LR7: Topock Gorge, San Bernardino County	Beginner	16.6 miles

Acknowledgments

I would like to thank my mother for encouraging me to write and my father for introducing me to the ocean. I would also like to thank my two sons, Matthew and Nathan, for their patience and understanding during the process of preparing this guidebook—I promise we will go surfing again. To Amie, a special thank you for all the encouragement and support you have given me.

To the rest of my family, friends and new acquaintances who accompanied me on my adventures (on and off the water) thank you: Chip, Carol, Kim, Heather, Justin, Brandon, Dave N., Dennis, Diane, Gary, Colette, Michael, Frank, Wayne, Tom and Dave from the Channel Islands National Park, Gigi, Paul, Jason, Jeff, Mike, Linda, Tim, Kelly, Pam, Sid, Warren, Dave, Angela, Tom, Ray, Mary, Susan, Judyth, Caroline, Tom, Paul, TC, Bonita, Tom, Len, Phil, Stu, and all my new CKF friends, the Island Packers crew, Bill, Demece, Joanne, Ed, Don, Les, Claudia, Jerry, Ben, Bill and to anyone else who I may have inadvertently neglected to mention, thank you.

Chapter 1

Planning the Trip

Thorough planning and preparation is essential for a safe and successful kayak tour. The following is a brief summary intended to introduce the reader to the factors that must be considered when preparing for a trip. The information provided should not be considered a complete treatment of the subject and should be supplemented with additional reading and training (see Selected References, at the end of this book). Courses on boating safety are available through the California Department of Boating and Waterways and the United States Coast Guard.

The Tour

Selecting an appropriate tour for you and for those in your group is the first step in planning your trip. Travel time, skill level, length of trip, points of interest, weather, and potential hazards must all be considered. Everyone in the group must be involved in the decision-making process and the degree of difficulty must be within the limits of the least-experienced paddler. Select a trip that fits your schedule and allows ample time for travel and set up. Identify at least one alternative tour in the event conditions are unfavorable for your first choice.

The Weather

The most important consideration when preparing for your trip is the weather. The weather can make the difference between an enjoyable adventure and a life-threatening disaster. With today's technology, there is an unlimited supply of information available to help you understand the weather. The Internet, television, radio, and the newspaper all provide a synopsis of local and worldwide weather conditions. Marine Weather Service Charts are published by the National Weather Service. Each chart lists the National Weather Service radio stations, office telephone numbers, and commercial radio broadcast stations that broadcast marine weather information along with their schedules.

The best times for kayaking in southern California are the summer and fall, although good weather can occur any time. During the summer, the weather is usually favorable and quite predictable. Seas are generally calm during the morning hours, but afternoon winds from the west measure 10-20 knots. Swells are normally small and out of the west or northwest with occasional strong south swells generated from South Pacific storms. These south swells normally last a day or two and primarily affect the south- and west-facing beaches. Water temperature during the summer varies from about 60 degrees Fahrenheit in the north to 70 degrees Fahrenheit in the south.

The fall is my favorite season for kayaking in California. The mornings are more likely to be clear and the winds are generally lighter than during the summer. While evenings can be cool, daytime temperatures are warm. Swells are usually small, and seas calm. As during the summer an occasional swell from the South Pacific or a hurricane off Central America can impact the south- and west-facing beaches. During the late fall, storm fronts coming from the Gulf of Alaska become increasingly frequent. Fall storms are usually weak and last only a day or two. Santa Ana winds are the most hazardous weather condition for kayakers during the fall. These gusty northeasterly winds mainly occur during the early evening and last for a few hours. The winds are often the strongest near shore at the head of a canyon. Santa Ana winds do not generate a strong swell but can create very choppy conditions which make paddling difficult. Santa Ana conditions can occur as often as four to six times a month. Water temperature during the fall varies from about 55 degrees Fahrenheit in the north to 65 degrees Fahrenheit in the south.

The winter months can be good for kayaking in Southern California but the conditions are less predictable. Powerful winter storms emanating from the Gulf of Alaska generate high winds and large swells that can last for several days at a time. Swells up to 20 feet high pound west- and northwest-facing beaches making launching or paddling a kayak impossible. During the peak of the storm, winds blow from the south or southeast. Strong northwest winds are likely during the 24 to 48 hours following the passage of a weather front. While adverse conditions can last for several days or even weeks at a time during the winter, calm warm weather perfect for kayaking can develop between the storms. The break between storms can last for a day or a month. Dense fog is not likely during the winter, but Santa Ana conditions can occur. Overnight trips are not recommended during the winter months. Water temperature during the winter varies from about 50 degrees Fahrenheit in the north to 60 degrees Fahrenheit in the south.

Northern storms also occur during the spring but usually with less frequency and for shorter duration than during the winter. Strong, gusty northwesterly winds are common during the spring. Morning hours can be suitable for kayaking but afternoons are often hazardous. South-facing beaches are usually the best locations for kayaking during the spring. Upwelling currents as a result of strong spring winds keep the water temperature cold. Fog and Santa Ana winds are unusual during the early spring. Water temperature during the spring varies from about 55 degrees Fahrenheit in the north to 65 degrees Fahrenheit in the south.

On the day preceding your paddle, obtain an accurate marine weather report. The information will help determine the most suitable location and time of day for your tour. If windy conditions or high seas are predicted, plan to paddle early in the morning in a protected cove, lake, or harbor. If calm conditions are predicted, an open-ocean paddle may be suitable. If storm advisories are reported, postpone your trip. On the morning of the paddle, listen to the weather report again, to hear whether the predictions have changed.

The Hazards

A kayak is a lightweight vessel that is sensitive to even the slightest change in conditions. An unforeseen ten-knot headwind can add hours to your planned travel time. A shift in the swell direction or an increase in the swell size can make landing at certain beaches impossible. In addition to obtaining an up-to-date weather forecast, the kayaker must be able to read the conditions of the water before leaving and while under way.

To effectively read the conditions, observe as much of your planned route as possible in advance. View the conditions at the launching and landing sites as well as at planned rest stops, points of interest, and prospective bail-out sites. Look for shallow reefs, dangerous headlands, thick kelpbeds that could impede your progress and always watch for fog. When paddling on a lake or in a confined harbor, be observant of boat traffic and follow the rules of the road. To gain a better perspective or your planned route, make your observations from a bluff top or from the top of a hill, as well as from the shoreline. Binoculars are useful when viewing from a distance.

When reading the waves, always be patient. It is important to observe the largest waves that you may expect to encounter. About 15 minutes should be enough time for accurate wave observations. It is also important to observe the time (period) between waves. How fast are the waves traveling? Are they closely spaced, or far apart? Are the waves plunging (breaking hard from top to bottom) or are they spilling (just breaking at the top and rolling toward the beach)? How much time will you have to launch or land between the largest waves? Watch carefully for waves that break on offshore reefs or sandbars and seaward traveling waves that may be reflected off cliffs or bulkheads. When the waves are big, select a lake or river tour or a tour within a harbor or protected bay.

Read the wind by studying its effects on the water and the environment. Use your binoculars and look far to sea. Both a darker shade of blue on the water and white caps are an indication of wind. Watch for sailboats. Are the sails full or are they limp? If there is fog or low clouds, can you observe its movement? Which direction is the fog moving? Is the surface of the ocean bumpy and choppy or is it flat and calm? Are the waves breaking on the beach in rapid succession (indicating nearby wind), or is there a long, regular interval between the waves? Which direction did the wind blow yesterday? Is today's weather similar to yesterday's? Plan your paddle so that you will have the wind coming from behind, and if possible avoid paddling during the afternoon when the wind is strongest.

Tidal information can be obtained from the weather report, a local newspaper, or a tide chart (available at most kayak shops and sporting-goods stores). There are usually two high tides and two low tides in a 24 hour period. Check the time of the high and low tides as well as the height of each tide. Plan your trip to have favorable tides for launching and landing and to avoid features along the route that may be exposed at low tide, such as shallow reefs, submerged offshore rocks and mud flats.

Currents are most noticeable in restricted waterways and estuaries, off headlands, near shallow reefs and sandbars, and between islands. The strength of the current dependents on the size of the tide, and the shape of the landform around or through which the water must move. Current tables can be used to predict the time, direction, and volume of flow in a given area. Some tables provide a factor for predicting the tidal change at other locations. In open waters the current direction can most easily be determined by observing movement of kelp. The long, trailing strands will point in the direction that the current is flowing. Currents can be both a help and a hazard for paddling. Whenever possible, plan your route to have a following current and to avoid headlands, reefs, and narrow channels where strong currents are known to exist.

Rip currents occur where incoming waves cause a temporary buildup of water near the shore. As the water escapes back to sea it causes a rip current. Rip currents usually occur along sandy shorelines with big waves. These currents are very strong, capable of carrying a swimmer quickly beyond the breakers. If you become trapped in a rip current, swim parallel to the shoreline until out of the current, then return to the beach. Rip currents are easily identified by their brown color and choppy, agitated water.

The water off the California coast is cold, especially during the spring and winter. Exposure to cold water is responsible for more sea kayaking deaths than any other cause. Hypothermia is the lowering of the body's inner core temperature. It occurs when the body loses more heat than it can produce. When exposed to cold, wet conditions or immersion in water, the body loses its ability to produce heat. The rate at which the body temperature falls is dependent on the water temperature, body type, movement, protective clothing, and the length of time in the water. For the average person, hypothermia begins after about 20 minutes in water that is 60 degrees Fahrenheit or less. To prevent hypothermia, the following precautions should be taken:

- Dress warmly with clothing, such as neoprene (wetsuit), that will cover your entire body and remain warm even when wet.
- Be sure that your boat is equipped with the necessary rescue equipment (see Equipment section of this book) and that you are familiar and comfortable with its use.
- Eat well and carry extra food.
- Head for shelter if you begin to get cold.
- Don't drink alcohol while paddling. It causes the body to lose heat faster.

Early recognition is important in the treatment of hypothermia. The symptoms include loss of mental ability, sluggish behavior, slurred speech, and violent shivering. If you suspect hypothermia, take the following steps immediately:

- Get the victim to shore.
- Remove wet clothing and replace with dry.
- Shelter the victim from the elements.
- Use body heat to warm the victim by getting inside a sleeping bag together. A core temperature increase of one degree Fahrenheit per hour is recommended.
- If the victim is conscious, administer warm fluids such as sweetened-tea, broth, or juice. Have the victim eat candy and other quick-energy foods. Do not give try to give food or drink to an unconscious victim.
- Get professional help as soon as possible.

Along the California coastline there are literally thousands of sea caves, many of which can be explored in a kayak. Some of the caves are only a few feet deep while others extend hundreds of feet and require a flashlight to explore. Use extreme caution when entering a sea cave. Never go alone, always wear a helmet, and be sure to carry a flashlight. Make sure you have plenty of headroom; even the wake of a passing boat or ship can create enough of a surge to close off a tight passageway or send you crashing into an overhead rock.

Locations for kayak surfing are identified for each tour. Kayak surfing is a fun but potentially hazardous sport. Shallow submerged rocks and strong currents are common. Always wear a helmet and a personal flotation device (PFD), and avoid all designated swimming and board surfing areas. Be considerate of others in the water, and remember a kayak weighs a lot more than a surfboard.

Lake and river kayaking have their own unique types of hazards. When paddling on a lake or river during the summer, hot weather must always be considered. Bring plenty of water and wear a broad brimmed hat for shade. Boat traffic often becomes congested so always follow the rules of the road. Watch for submerged rocks, snags and low overhanging brush. Winds are usually gusty and unpredictable. Whenever possible, plan your route to have a following wind. Although waves are not a hazard on lakes, chop is. If you will be exploring the shoreline, watch for natural hazards such as rattlesnakes, ticks, insects, and poison oak. Some lakes and rivers are in remote areas where mountain lions are occasionally observed. Although the likelihood of encountering an aggressive lion is rare, it is a good idea to never hike alone and young children should be closely supervised at all times.

The Float Plan

After you decide where and when to go on your tour, it's time to prepare a float plan. A float plan, the equivalent of an airplane pilot's flight plan, includes the information that would assist a rescue operation. The float plan should include:

- Time and location of departure, route, destination, intermediate checkpoints.
- When you should be considered overdue.
- Names, addresses, and phone numbers of all the members of the group.
- A brief description of your boats and the equipment for signaling and self-rescue.
- Name and phone number of who to notify in the event you are overdue.

The float plan should be "filed" with a family member or other responsible party.

The Kayak

Selecting the right kayak depends on the type of paddling you intend to do. As a general rule, longer and sleeker boats are better for open-ocean paddling and shorter boats offer more maneuverability for the surf, sea caves and near-shore conditions. Fiberglass and kevlar boats are lighter and faster; however, polyethylene boats are more durable and well suited for use in a rocky environment. There are hundreds of designs to choose from, and your local kayak dealer will be able help you select the right boat.

The Equipment

A well-equipped kayak is essential for a safe and enjoyable trip. Your equipment must include everything necessary to contend with any situation that may arise. Obviously the equipment you carry will depend on the type of boat you are paddling, length of the trip, and the conditions you may encounter. To be sure that you have everything you need, develop a checklist to keep with your kayak. Mount the list on the inside of your hatch cover or other convenient location. Equipment can be divided into essential and optional items. Never paddle without the essential equipment. Following is a sample checklist of essential equipment:

personal flotation device (PFD)	wet suit/booties	sunscreen
helmet	repair kit	tide and current tables
paddle	compass	spare clothes
spray skirt*	chart	flashlight or headlamp
paddle (and spare)	navigation gear	tow rope
self-rescue gear	weather radio	knife
signaling device	drinking water/food	paddle leash
hand pump and sponge*	first aid kit	spray jacket
watch	sunglasses	hat
binoculars		

 * open deck boats only

Navigation

Navigation is the process of planning a route, knowing where you have been, where you are, and where you are going. Anyone planning an open-ocean paddle should be familiar with the principles of navigation. Basic navigation is included in most beginner kayaking courses. More advanced courses are offered through the Coast Guard and various other maritime agencies and groups. The *Fundamentals of Kayak Navigation*, by David Burch, is an excellent resource.

The most common method for coastal kayaking navigation is piloting. Piloting is the use of visual landmarks to establish your location and route. The simplest method of piloting is line of sight, without the use of a compass or chart.

Unfortunately, landmarks are not always recognizable at distances of one to two miles or during foggy or hazy conditions. To keep from getting lost during conditions of limited visibility requires a method of navigation known as dead reckoning. Dead reckoning involves the use of speed, time, and compass course to plot your position. Most navigation is actually a combination of piloting and dead reckoning.

Plotting a course while under way in a kayak is not practical; it should be done before launching. Routes should be plotted between prominent headlands or other visible landmarks. Winds, tides, and potential hazards such as submerged rocks must always be taken into consideration when planning your route. Whenever possible paddle with the current and avoid headwinds.

Along the California coast this usually means paddling from north to south. To maintain a set course when paddling across the wind or current, you must compensate for drift by heading the boat at a slight angle, known as a ferry angle, into the wind or current. The stronger the crosswind or current, the greater the ferry angle and the paddling speed required to compensate for drift. The basic navigation tools include: compass, chart case, chart, divider, parallel rule or protractor, grease pencil, tide and current tables, and watch.

California Boating Law

California Boating Law applies to the operation of all types of vessels (boats, ships, personal watercraft, etc.) on all waters within US territorial limits. The navigational rules, commonly called the rules of the road govern the operation of all vessels. Although vessels under manual propulsion, such as kayaks, are generally favored with the right of way, paddlers must be familiar with the rules of the road in order to avoid collisions. The basic rules of the road are as follows:

- Vessels under power yield to vessels under sail which yield to manually propelled vessels.
- When meeting head-on, vessels shall pass to the right of each other.
- When meeting at an angle, the vessel on the right has the right of way.
- A vessel overtaking another vessel from astern shall keep out of the way of the vessel being overtaken.
- Vessels shall keep to the right in narrow channels.
- Small vessels shall not impede the passage of large vessels when operating in a narrow channel.
- Vessels shall not tie up to navigational buoys or markers.

The waters of the United States are marked for safe passage by a system of buoys. The system uses an arrangement of colors, shapes, numbers, and lights to indicate the side on which a buoy should be passed when proceeding in a given direction. The characteristics are determined by the position of the buoy with respect to the navigable channels as the channels are entered from seaward. "Red right returning" is a saying used by mariners as a reminder to keep red-colored buoys on the starboard (right) side when entering a harbor. Likewise green buoys are kept on the port (left) side when entering a harbor. The standard buoy markings when proceeding into a harbor or upstream in a river are as follows:

- Port-hand buoys are painted green, odd-numbered, with green lights.

- Starboard-hand buoys are painted red, even-numbered, with red lights.
- Mid-channel buoys have red and white vertical stripes.

Navigational signals are used for vessels in sight of each other to indicate the intended course for safe navigation. Kayakers are not required to carry navigational signaling devices but should be aware of their use. The following are the standard signals:

- One short blast of the signaling device indicates an intention to turn the vessel to starboard (right).
- Two short blasts of the signaling device indicates an intention to turn the vessel to port (left).
- Three short blasts of the signaling device indicates the vessel's engines are going astern (in reverse).
- Five or more short, rapid blasts of the signaling device indicate a danger signal.
- A prolonged blast of four to six seconds indicates a situation of restricted visibility or maneuverability.

Running lights are required for all vessels operating between sunset and sunrise and during periods of restricted visibility. Vessels under paddle or oar must have, ready at hand, an electric torch or waterproof flashlight showing a white light which must be exhibited in sufficient time to prevent a collision.

Manually propelled boats of any size are required to carry visual distress signaling devices only for travel at night. All visible distress-signaling devices must be Coast Guard approved, readily accessible, and in serviceable condition. The absence of legally required daytime distress signals does not mean they are unnecessary. Hand-held flares, smoke canisters, dye marker, and a "May Day" signal all provide a clear signal of distress. The accepted "May Day" signal for a kayaker is to hold your paddle horizontally and move it repeatedly up and down. To report an emergency, the Coast Guard can be reached any time on VHF radio, channel 16.

The Environment

California's coastline, lakes, and rivers are areas of unparalleled beauty blessed with a rich diversity of plants, animals, and natural resources. Each year, millions of people visit these fragile environments. With the increased popularity of kayaking, many areas that were previously inaccessible to the public are now visited often. By following the guidelines listed below, you can help preserve these priceless resources and protect the wildlife for future generations to enjoy:

- Under federal law it is illegal to disturb and/or harass marine mammals. Harassment may be any action that modifies the behavior of the animal. Try to stay 50 to 100 yards away from all animals whether in the water or on shore. If they look your way and appear disturbed, you are too close and should move quietly away. Disturbed animals may leave the area temporarily or permanently. Sometimes curious animals will swim up to you. Remain calm and avoid quick movements or actions that could disturb them.
- Avoid areas such as offshore rocks, sea caves, or secluded beaches where seals, sea lions or other pinnipeds are pupping. Disturbed pinnipeds may abandon their pups.
- Try to remain at least 100 yards from any marine mammal haul-out. Sea lions and harbor seals haul out on beaches to absorb heat from the sun to warm their bodies. Rest periods are important for their energy budget.
- Do not disturb nesting or roosting sea birds. When adults leave the nest the eggs may overheat in the sun or be eaten by gulls or ravens.
- Do not disturb or touch a stranded or injured animal. Notify the marine-mammal protection center in your area.
- Be observant and step lightly when exploring tide pools. Don't pull animals off the rocks. Tide-pool animals are easily damaged and may die from being handled. Many tide pools are protected by law, and removing any plant or animal from them is illegal.
- Do not feed native wildlife.
- Pack out all of your trash and pick up trash that you may find. Leave the area cleaner than you found it.
- A valid California State fishing license is required to fish.
- Abide by all California Department of Fish and Game regulations and all other posted regulations.

For more information

Channel Islands National Marine Sanctuary (805) 966-7107
Monterey Bay National Marine Sanctuary (408) 647-4201
Marine Mammal Center Hotline (408) 633-6298
California Department of Fish and Game, Marine Resources Division (916) 653-6281
National Marine Fisheries Service (562) 980-4050

MAP LEGEND

Kayak Tours

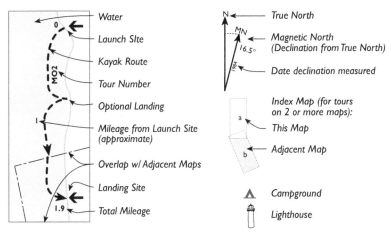

- Water
- Launch Site
- Kayak Route
- Tour Number
- Optional Landing
- Mileage from Launch Site (approximate)
- Overlap w/ Adjacent Maps
- Landing Site
- Total Mileage

- True North
- Magnetic North (Declination from True North)
- Date declination measured
- Index Map (for tours on 2 or more maps):
- This Map
- Adjacent Map
- ▲ Campground
- Lighthouse

Water & Land

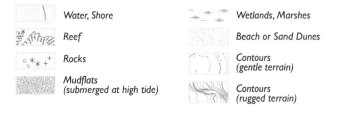

- Water, Shore
- Reef
- Rocks
- Mudflats (submerged at high tide)

- Wetlands, Marshes
- Beach or Sand Dunes
- Contours (gentle terrain)
- Contours (rugged terrain)

Highways and Roads

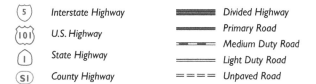

- (5) Interstate Highway
- (101) U.S. Highway
- (1) State Highway
- (S1) County Highway

- Divided Highway
- Primary Road
- Medium Duty Road
- Light Duty Road
- ==== Unpaved Road

Tour Location Maps

- **ORI** ☐ Tours in This Chapter
- LA8 ⬚ Tours in Other Chapters
- Lakes, Ocean

- Freeway
- Highway
- Local Road
- ◯ ◦ Cities & Towns
- County Line, State Line

Monterey County Tours

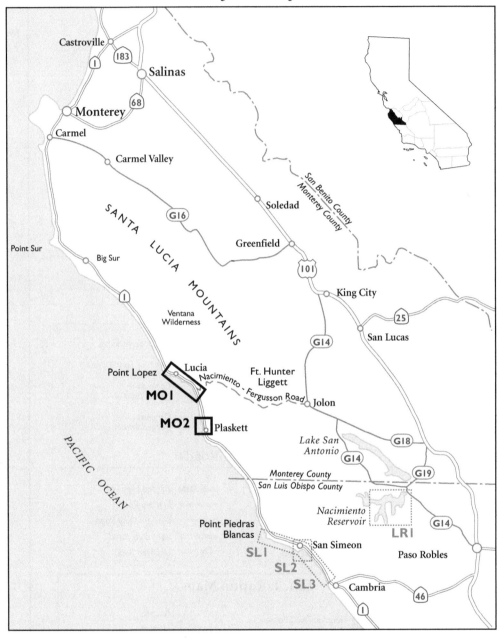

Tour	Skill Level	Length
MO1: Mill Creek to Lopez Point	Intermediate	10.5 miles
MO2: Sand Dollar Beach to Jade Cove	Advanced	2.2 miles

Chapter 2

Monterey County

The Big Sur coastline is a kayaking frontier. It is an area visited by many but explored by few. Each adventure to this rugged coastline is a unique and exciting experience filled with new challenges and rewards.

My first kayaking trip to Big Sur was in 1995. I had recently met some new friends who had expressed an interest in the area but knew nothing about it. I had been on numerous surfing and fishing expeditions to Big Sur but never had dared a trip in my kayak. I met my friends in San Simeon and we caravaned the rest of the way up the coast. It was late summer and there was a thick morning haze. As we meandered along Highway 1, we could periodically catch a glimpse of gray ocean hundreds of feet below us. I was relieved to see that the waves appeared to be small and there was no wind. After traveling for about an hour we finally reached our destination, a launch spot that I knew was used by local dory fishermen. It is one of the few locations on the Big Sur coast that is sheltered from the waves and accessible by car. The fog was beginning to clear and the gray tones that shrouded the surroundings were soon replaced by a spectrum of bright colors.

I was apprehensive as I carried my kayak to the water. For years I had dreamed about kayaking this coast and now that it was becoming a reality I was actually fearful; fearful of the unknown. My heart was pounding as I took a deep breath and launched through the waves. When I finally paused to look back, I was stunned by what I saw. The fear that seemed so prevalent a moment ago was overcome with awe by the spectacular beauty that surrounded me. My heart was still pounding but more from excitement than from fear.

I waited for my friends to breach the waves and then we headed north. As we paddled along I was amazed by what I saw. Towering coastal mountains, forests of kelp, and crystal clear water that seemed to capture the suns rays in the endless abyss. What struck me most was the magnitude of everything around me. I had never been in a place where I felt so small and overwhelmed by my surroundings.

As we continued, my fear diminished. A harbor seal poked his large gray head through the kelp and looked at me reassuringly as if to say "Don't worry, everything is OK." I realized that I had nothing to fear but fear itself. I had a peaceful feeling of oneness with the environment.

I learned a lot that day. A lot about myself and a lot about the world in which we live. It was a day I will always remember.

— *Mill Creek, September 10, 1995*

TOUR M01 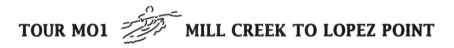 MILL CREEK TO LOPEZ POINT

Tour Details

Skill level:	Intermediate
Trip length/type:	10.5 miles; round trip; open-ocean; four to five hours
Chart/map:	NOAA Chart #18700; USGS *Lopez Point* and *Cape San Martin* 7.5 min series

Summary

Aside from the Channel Islands, the Big Sur coastline is perhaps the most secluded and pristine section of coastline in California. Cone Peak, which stands at an elevation of over 5000 feet, provides the backdrop for this magnificent tour through sea caves and glistening kelp forests.

How to get there

To reach the launch site exit, Highway 1 at the Mill Creek Picnic Area, which is one-quarter mile south of Nacimiento Fergusson Road. Parking, restrooms and picnic facilities are available. Fee.

Camping

Camping is available at Limekiln Campground located on Highway 1 approximately two and one-half miles north of Mill Creek Picnic Area. For camping reservations, call ParkNet (800) 444-7275. Camping is also available at Kirk Creek Campground, on Highway 1 approximately one mile north of Mill Creek, and at Plaskett Creek Campground, on Highway 1, approximately five miles south of Mill Creek. Individual campsites are available on a first-come/first-served basis at Kirk Creek and Plaskett Creek. For information call (805) 995-1761 or (805) 995-1976. For information and reservations for group camping, call (800) 280-CAMP.

Hazards

Do not attempt this paddle if strong winds or large waves are predicted. Stay clear of offshore rocks and shoals. Thick fog or Santa Ana winds can occur at any time of the year. Wear a helmet and PFD, and carry a waterproof flashlight when exploring the caves.

Public access

Kirk Creek Campground and Limekiln Campground. Most of the land between Highway 1 and the water is privately owned, very steep, and inaccessible. This tour is within the Monterey Bay National Marine Sanctuary.

Kayak surfing

This section of coast is not noted for kayak surfing. Occasionally there are ridable waves on the beach below the Kirk Creek Campground.

Launching

A short dirt pathway leads from the Mill Creek Picnic Area to the beach. The best place to launch is from the sandy cove just north of the parking lot. The waves are usually small and break close to shore but a surf launch may be necessary.

Tour description

From the launch site at Mill Creek, follow the coastline northwest. The marine terrace is very narrow and the mountains rise abruptly to an elevation of nearly one mile. Highway 1, the only major road in the area, can be seen winding its way precariously along the steep hillside. The north-facing mountain slopes are forested with coastal redwoods, and year-round streams flow from many of the steep, narrow canyons. The beach is narrow and rocky with occasional sandy pocket beaches in the sheltered coves. Just north of Mill Creek and about one-quarter mile offshore are a thick kelp bed and a shallow reef with breaking waves. The water is usually extremely clear, and this is a favorite spot for scuba divers. The fishing is excellent, with gopher cod, ling

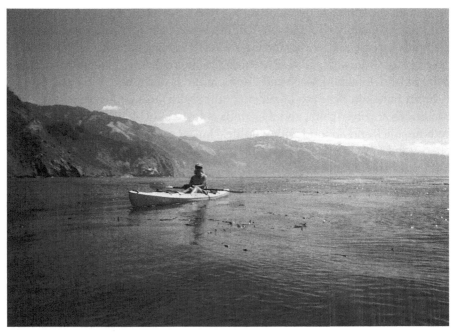

Calm water near Limekiln Beach

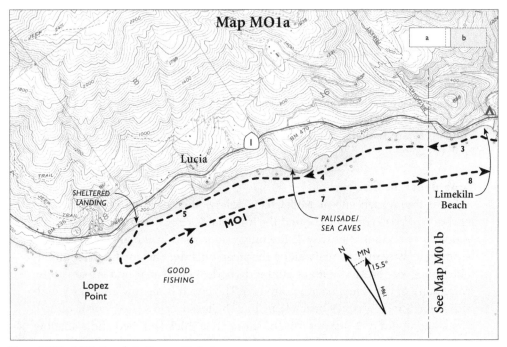

Tour MO1: Mill Creek to Lopez Point

cod, and cabezon the normal "catch of the day." Kirk Creek Campground can be seen on the bluff top overlooking the reef.

At approximately two and one-half miles is an abrupt, rocky headland. On the southeast side of the headland is a sheltered landing site with a cobble beach. Several large sea caves, accessible during calm conditions, extend through the point of land. Limekiln Beach and Campground is northwest of the point.

From Limekiln Beach to Lopez Point the shore faces almost due south. Sea conditions are often calm, and the winds occasionally blow offshore. The kelp beds are thick and abound with wildlife. Harbor seals, California sea lions, sea otters, and a wide variety of shore birds can be observed year-round. California gray whales visit the area during winter and spring.

At approximately four miles is a high rocky palisade. The towering vertical cliffs drop straight into the sea. Several massive sea caves have been eroded in the dense rock by the powerful waves. Use extreme caution when approaching the caves; the current can be very strong and the waves surge with tremendous force. Do not attempt to paddle into the caves unless conditions are very calm. The smooth walls of the caverns are bright red and shine like glass. The water is deep and clear and the tidepools are filled with an abundance of sea life.

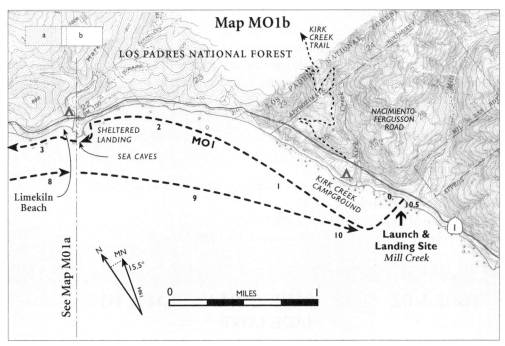

Tour MO1 (continued)

From the palisade to Lopez Point is approximately one and one-half miles. Perched high on the bluff just west of the palisade is the community of Lucia, which consists of a restaurant, gas station, store, and motel. The wind and waves are generally calm in the shelter of the Lopez Point. The shoreline is narrow and strewn with boulders and cobbles, but landing is possible at several locations. Offshore, the kelpbeds are thick and fishing is excellent. During spring, Lopez Point is an excellent location for viewing California gray whales on their annual migration from Alaska to Baja California. Near the point is a trail that leads from the beach to the bluff top, but the property is private and trespassing is prohibited.

Proceed cautiously when approaching Lopez Point; the waves can be unpredictable, the reefs treacherous, and the currents strong. Paddling north of Lopez Point is not recommended unless you are well prepared and have experience paddling on the Big Sur coast. From Lopez Point return to Mill Creek.

Landing

Land in the cove to the north of the parking lot at the Mill Creek Picnic Area.

What to do afterward

There are numerous hiking trails in the Los Padres National Forest and the Ventana Wilderness. Trail guides are available at the ranger station at Pacific Valley just north of the Plaskett Creek Campground. Mission San Antonio, one of the original California missions, is approximately 15 miles to the east, just off the Nacimiento Fergusson Road.

Alternate tour: Tour SL2

For more information

The Los Padres National Forest, Monterey District (408) 385-5434
Big Sur Station (408) 667-2315
U.S. Coast Guard, Monterey (408) 647-7303
Monterey Bay National Marine Sanctuary (408) 647-4201

TOUR MO2 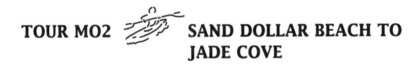 SAND DOLLAR BEACH TO JADE COVE

Tour Details

Skill level:	Advanced (can be suitable for intermediate level during calm conditions)
Trip length/type:	2.2 miles; round trip;open-ocean; one to two hours
Chart/map:	NOAA Chart #18700; USGS *Cape San Martin* 7.5 min series

Summary

A beautiful white-sand beach with great waves for kayak surfing, large off-shore rocks, kelp forests, and sea otters are all included on this Big Sur coastal adventure.

How to get there

To reach the launch site, exit Highway 1 at the Sand Dollar Beach Picnic Area about five miles south of Nacimiento Fergusson Road. Parking, restrooms, and picnic facilities are available. Fee.

Camping

Camping is available at Limekiln Campground on Highway 1, approximately ten miles north of Sand Dollar Beach. For camping reservations, call ParkNet (800) 444-7275. Camping is also available at Kirk Creek Campground on Highway 1, approximately eight miles north of Sand Dollar Beach and at Plaskett Creek Campground directly across Highway 1 from Sand Dollar Beach. Individual campsites are available on a first-come/first-served basis at Kirk Creek and Plaskett Creek. For information call (805) 995-1761 or (805) 995-1976. For information and reservations for group camping, call (800) 280-CAMP.

Hazards

Do not attempt this paddle if strong winds or large swells are predicted. Stay clear of offshore rocks and shoals. Thick fog or Santa Ana winds can occur at any time of the year.

Public access

The bluff is very steep and the beach is mostly inaccessible. There is a dirt path leading to Jade Cove, but the waves are usually large and landing is not suggested. This tour is within the Monterey Bay National Marine Sanctuary.

Kayak surfing

Sand Dollar Beach is noted for its good waves.

Launching

Kayaks must be carried about one hundred yards across the marine terrace and down a long flight of stairs to the beach. If the waves are small, and you are experienced at surf launching, launch from the beach directly in front of the stairway. Otherwise, the best place to launch is in the lee of the large offshore rock at the south end of the beach. Launching from Sand Dollar Beach should not be considered when the waves are large.

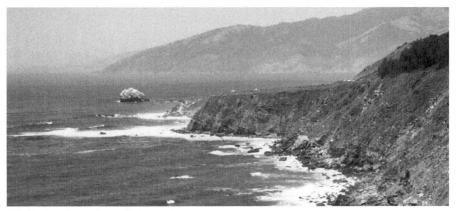

Plaskett Rock and Lopez Point

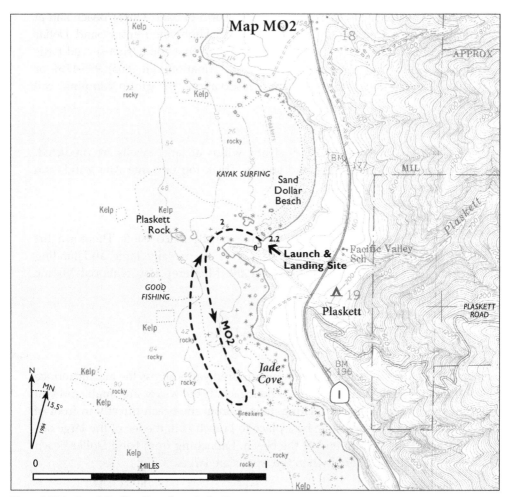

Map MO2

Tour MO2: Sand Dollar Beach to Jade Cove

Tour description

During calm conditions there are several large offshore rocks to explore in the cove at Sand Dollar Beach. From Sand Dollar Beach, proceed south around the point at the south end of the bay, staying inside of Plaskett Rock. This section of coast is very exposed to wind and waves, so even under the best conditions it's impossible to paddle very close to shore. Offshore the kelp forests are thick and wildlife is abundant. California sea lions, harbor seals, and sea otters are commonly seen. Sea otters, with their reddish brown to black fur, are easy to spot as they swim and play in the kelp beds. The sea otter is well known for its ability to use rock tools to assist in feeding. While swimming on its back, the otter will use a rock to break open the hard protective shell of an abalone, crab, or other shellfish which it holds on its chest. Because the sea otter does not have a thick layer of blubber to protect it from the cold like most marine mammals, it must consume tremendous amounts of food to maintain its body temperature; up to 2.5 tons of food annually. For its thick, soft fur, the sea otter was hunted to near extinction. From the mid-1700s to early 1900, perhaps over a million sea otters were killed by Russian, American, and European fur traders. Today the sea otter is protected by state and federal law. Most of the southern sea otters live within the California Sea Otter Game Refuge, which extends from the Carmel River in Monterey County to Santa Rosa Creek in San Luis Obispo County.

Jade Cove is about one mile south of Sand Dollar Beach. A trail can be seen leading from the bluff top to the water's edge. The cove is small and conditions are generally too rough to land. From Jade Cove, return to Sand Dollar Beach.

Landing

If the waves are small and you are experienced at surf landings, land on the beach near the base of the stairway to the beach. Otherwise land in the lee of the offshore rock at the south end of Sand Dollar Beach.

What to do afterward

Sand Dollar Beach has picnic facilities and several miles of scenic, bluff-top hiking and biking trails; fishing is excellent. Jade Cove is accessible from Highway 1. Park at the Jade Cove sign and follow the trail to the beach. Jade Cove is one of the few places in the world that the semi-precious nephite jade can be found. Removal of jade found above the high-tide level is prohibited by law.

Alternate tour: Tour SL2

For more information

Los Padres National Forest, Monterey District (408) 385-5434
Big Sur Station (408) 667-2315
US Coast Guard (408) 647-7303
Monterey Bay National Marine Sanctuary (408) 647-4201

San Luis Obispo County Tours

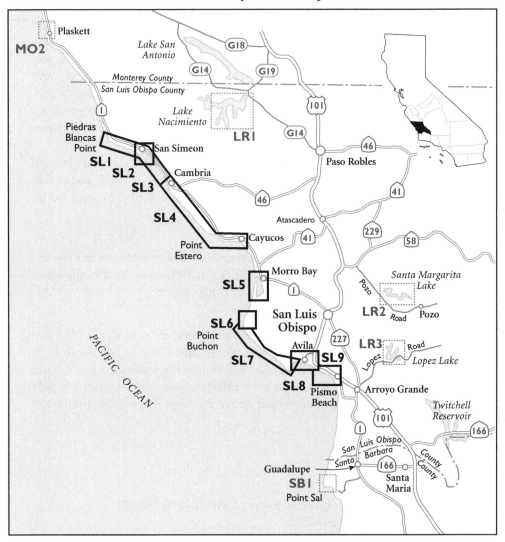

Tour		Skill Level	Length
SL1:	Piedras Blancas Point to San Simeon Cove	Intermediate	8.5 miles
SL2:	San Simeon Cove	Beginner	1.5 miles
SL3:	San Simeon Cove to Leffingwell Landing	Advanced	6.0 miles
SL4:	Shammel Park to Cayucos Pier	Advanced	17.2 miles
SL5:	Morro Bay Harbor and Estuary	Beginner	11.3 miles
SL6:	Montana de Oro	Advanced	4.1 miles
SL7:	Spooner's Cove to Olde Port Beach	Advanced	17.0 miles
SL8:	Olde Port Beach to Pirate's Cove	Beginner	9.3 miles
SL9:	Shell Beach	Beginner	4.4 miles

Chapter 3

San Luis Obispo County

Paddling in the calm waters of the bay was a nice change from the open ocean. With the aid of the outgoing tide, our kayaks glided effortlessly past the restaurants and shops along the Embarcadero. The familiar smell of fish and chips reminded me that it was almost lunch time. It was a cool, drizzly day and the people looked warm and cozy sitting at their brightly lit tables.

Ahead, Morro Rock stood like a sentinel guarding the entrance to the bay. Its peak was shrouded in a misty fog. A hungry sea otter, busy munching on a large spider crab, floated past us on his back.

Low tide was still an hour away and we didn't want to return against the tidal current so we decided to go for a hike. We crossed the channel to the sand spit, pulled our kayaks onto the dry sand and headed out across the dunes. The wind was beginning to blow and it became rather chilly. Fortunately we had plenty of clothes to keep us warm.

The waves were pounding on the unprotected outer beach. A couple of lonely surf fishermen stood motionless next to their poles as if frozen in time. We collected some beautiful sand dollars and some interesting sculptured pieces of driftwood then found a nice protected spot to have lunch. We were really hungry and everything tasted great.

By the time we got back to our kayaks, the ebb tide was upon us. We made good time as we headed for the estuary, weaving our way in and out of the boats lying at anchor. A fishing boat passed, followed by swarm of noisy sea gulls frantically competing for leftovers.

The Morro Bay Estuary is a special place that provides a safe habitat for dozens of endangered and protected species. We meandered through the narrow tidal channels bordered by thick marsh grass. A small fish jumped and a tall, blue heron stood motionless in the shallow water. The heron reminded me of the fishermen we had seen on the beach. The estuary was so peaceful and quiet, but very much alive with wildlife.

— Morro Bay, February 14, 1995

TOUR SL1 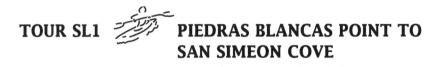 PIEDRAS BLANCAS POINT TO SAN SIMEON COVE

Tour Details

Skill level:	Intermediate
Trip length/type:	8.5 miles; one-way; open-ocean; cove; three to four hours
Chart/map:	NOAA Chart #18700; USGS *Piedras Blancas* and *San Simeon* 7.5 min series

Summary

The famous Hearst Castle (Hearst San Simeon State Historical Monument) overlooks this relatively calm and protected section of coast. Along the route you will pass an elephant seal colony, explore tide pools and sea caves, and relax on a warm, sandy beach. If you bring your fishing pole, plan on a fish dinner.

How to get there

To reach the launch site exit Highway 1 at Piedras Blancas Point, about five miles west of William R. Hearst Memorial State Beach in San Simeon. There are two parking lots about one and one-half miles east of Piedras Blancas Point. Park in the easternmost lot. No facilities are provided. No fee.

To reach the landing site, exit Highway 1 at William R. Hearst Memorial State Beach. Enter the State Beach and park in the lower parking lot adjacent to the beach. Restrooms, picnic facilities, and telephones are provided. Fee.

Camping

Tent and RV campsites are available at San Simeon State Park on Highway 1 about six miles southeast of William R. Hearst Memorial State Beach. For camping reservations, call ParkNet (800) 444-7275.

Hazards

Winds usually blow offshore (from land to sea), which keeps the sea relatively flat. Piedras Blancas Point buffers the northwesterly swells; however, don't paddle too far offshore on windy days. Returning to shore can be difficult with a strong headwind. Watch for shallow, submerged rocks when exploring the tidepools. Wear a helmet and PFD, and carry a waterproof flashlight when exploring the caves.

Public access

Other than designated public viewpoints, most of the coastal land between Highway 1 and the water is owned by the Hearst Corporation. The beach at San Simeon Cove is public and accessible through the William R. Hearst Memorial State Beach. This tour is within the Monterey Bay National Marine Sanctuary.

Kayak surfing

Good waves for kayak surfing can be found at Arroyo Laguna Creek, about three and one-half miles east of Piedras Blancas Point.

Launching

Launch from the sand beach just west of the easternmost parking lot about one and one-half miles south of Piedras Blancas Point. The waves are usually small and break near the shore, but a surf launch may be necessary.

Tour description

Paddle beyond the breakers and head toward Piedras Blancas lighthouse, about one and one-half miles west. A large colony of Northern elephant seals inhabit the coves between the launch site and the lighthouse. The males grow up to 14 feet in length and weigh as much as 5000 pounds. The elephant seal derives its name from its large size and the male's elephant-like snout. Females are much smaller and lack the large snout, but like the males are a brownish-gray color. Elephant seals are deep divers, second only to sperm whales. As nocturnal feeders, elephant seals feed primarily on rays, rock fish, squid, and small sharks. Keep a safe distance from these creatures; they can be quite aggressive, especially when protecting their young.

Piedras Blancas ("white rocks" in Spanish) was named by the explorer Juan Rodriguez Cabrillo in 1542. The headland is relatively low-lying, with several large, guano-covered rocks a short distance offshore. To the east of the point, the water is sheltered from the wind and waves; fishing and scuba diving are excellent. Otters, harbor seals, and sea lions inhabit the thick beds of giant kelp, and during winter and spring California gray whales are commonly seen. In 1864 a lookout was constructed on Piedras Blancas Point to alert whalers in the nearby whaling station at San Simeon of approaching whales. In 1874 the lookout was replaced with a permanent lighthouse. In 1949, the original lens and iron lantern house were replaced by an automated beacon. Both the lens and lantern house are on display in the nearby town of Cambria, next to the Veteran's Memorial Building on Main Street.

From Piedras Blancas Point, head east past the launching site toward San Simeon Point, about five miles southeast. San Simeon Point is vegetated with

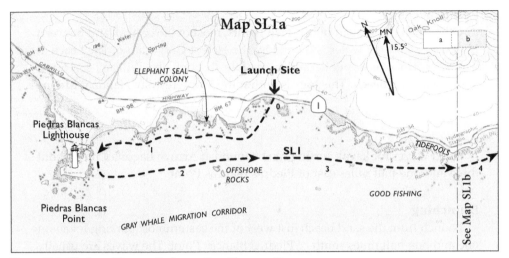

Tour SL1: Piedras Blancas Point to San Simeon Cove

large cypress trees and is usually clearly visible from the water. Two large rocks about one-half mile offshore from the launch site are a favorite haul-out for harbor seals and sea lions as well as a rookery for cormorants. Keep a safe distance from the rocks to avoid disturbing the animals or getting caught by a sneaker wave.

The shoreline between Piedras Blancas Point and San Simeon Point consists of a wide, flat rock shelf which is exposed at low tide. The shallow tide pools are inhabited by a variety of organisms including snails, crabs, mussels, anenomes, urchins, limpets, abalone, octopuses, eels, barnacles, and sea stars. The waves are generally calm, and landing is possible at several locations. Offshore, the thick beds of giant kelp provide the perfect habitat for a wide variety of rock fish such as gopher cod, ling cod, cabezon, and china cod. A kayak, with its shallow draft and good maneuverability, is the perfect fishing boat for these conditions.

To the east of the tide pools is Arroyo Laguna Beach, a popular wind-surfing spot. Waves usually break on the beach and it is not a good landing site. At the east end of Arroyo Laguna Beach are two small sheltered coves, which offer a protected landing under most conditions. Both coves are popular harbor seal haul-outs.

During the afternoon, very choppy conditions can be encountered on the west side of San Simeon Point. Remain a safe distance offshore and watch for shallow submerged rocks when rounding the point. Within San Simeon Cove the wind and sea are generally calm. Explore the sea caves and secluded pocket beaches along the rocky shoreline at the west end of the cove. The beautiful sand beach to the west of the pier is warm and sheltered.

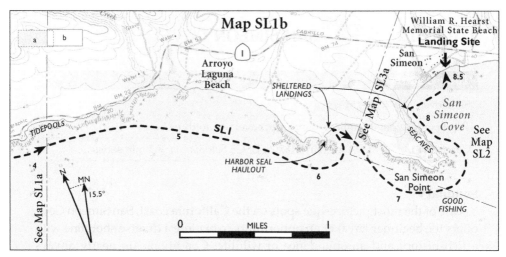

Tour SL1 (continued)

Landing

Land at the beach just west of the pier at William R. Hearst Memorial State Beach. Conditions are usually calm but a surf landing may be necessary.

What to do afterward

Hearst Castle is across Highway 1 from San Simeon Cove. Food and snacks are available at the Sebastian's General Store, one of the oldest continuously operating stores in California. The building was originally part of the whaling station that operated on San Simeon Point during the 1800s.

Alternate tour: SL2

For more information

William R. Hearst Memorial State Beach (805) 927-2068
US Coast Guard (805)772-2167
Monterey Bay National Marine Sanctuary (408) 647-4201

TOUR SL2 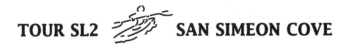 SAN SIMEON COVE

Tour Details

Skill level:	Beginner
Trip length/type:	1.5 miles; round-trip; cove; two to three hours
Chart/map:	NOAA Chart #18700; USGS *San Simeon* 7.5 min series

Summary

One of the most picturesque spots on the California coast, San Simeon Cove offers the beginner kayaker an opportunity to explore a diverse shoreline with a rich history and an abundance of wildlife. Conditions are nearly always calm on this two-to-three mile trip.

How to get there

To reach the launch site exit Highway 1 at William R. Hearst Memorial State Beach in San Simeon. Enter the State Beach and park in the lower parking lot adjacent to the beach. Restrooms, picnic facilities, and telephones are provided. Fee.

Camping

Tent and RV campsites are available at San Simeon State Park on Highway 1 about six miles southeast of William R. Hearst Memorial State Beach. For camping reservations, call ParkNet (800) 444-7275.

Hazards

San Simeon Point offers protection from the prevailing northwest wind and swells. Rough conditions can occur during winter storms when the wind blows from the south. Wear a helmet and PFD, and carry a waterproof flashlight when exploring the caves.

Public access

The beach at San Simeon Cove is public and accessible through the State Park. San Simeon Point is privately owned. This tour is within the Monterey Bay National Marine Sanctuary.

Kayak surfing

Waves are small and not suitable for kayak surfing in San Simeon Cove.

Launching

Launch from the beach just west of the pier at William R. Hearst Memorial State Beach. Conditions are usually calm but a surf launching may be necessary.

Tour description

From the launch site, follow the shoreline towards the rocky cliffs at the west end of the beach. On the low bluff above the beach are several homes and warehouses built by the Hearst family. The sea is usually calm, and a warm breeze blows gently off the land. Because of its ideal weather, San Simeon Cove is one of the most popular beaches in San Luis Obispo County.

From the west end of the beach, follow the rocky bluff toward the point. Explore the many sea caves and small, secluded coves along the way. The bright green Monterey pines atop the bluff provide a brilliant contrast to the deep-blue water of the cove. It's easy to imagine what it must have been like during the 1920s and 1930s when famous film stars visited William Hearst at his castle on the hill.

Approach the point carefully. Large waves build suddenly and break on the submerged rocks just offshore. During very calm conditions, a landing can be made at the beach just inside the point. If you enjoy fishing, try your luck in the kelp beds off the end of the point. All you need is a good pole equipped with 30-pound test line, a rock-cod jig, and an eight-ounce sinker.

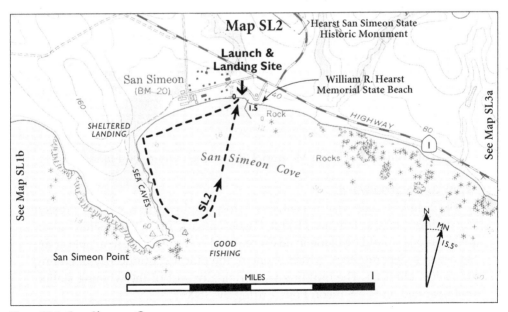

Tour SL2: San Simeon Cove

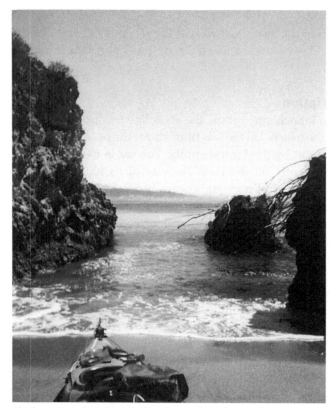

Explore the secluded pocket beaches in San Simeon Cove

With a little patience and some squid for bait you'll have dinner in no time. Cabezon and rock cod are the usual catch of the day.

From San Simeon Point return to the launch site by paddling directly across the bay, or head back to the beach and spend the rest of the afternoon enjoying the warm sunshine and beautiful scenery.

Landing
Land at William R. Hearst Memorial State Beach where you launched.

What to do afterward
The Hearst Castle visitor center is across Highway 1 from San Simeon Cove. Tours of the famous Hearst Castle embark from the visitor center. Reservations should be made in advance. Food and snacks are available at the Sebastian's General Store, which is one of the oldest continuously operating stores in California. The building was originally part of the whaling station that operated on San Simeon Point during the 1800s.

Alternate tour: SL5

For more information

William R. Hearst Memorial State Beach (805) 927-2068

US Coast Guard (805) 772-2167

Monterey Bay National Marine Sanctuary (408) 647-4201

TOUR SL3 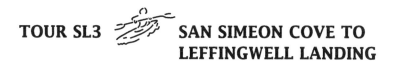 SAN SIMEON COVE TO LEFFINGWELL LANDING

Tour Details	
Skill level:	Advanced
Trip length/type:	6.0 miles; one-way; open ocean; three to four hours
Chart/map:	NOAA Chart #18700; USGS *San Simeon* and *Pico Creek* 7.5 min series

Summary

Sea otters and harbor seals will provide entertainment as you meander through the thick beds of giant kelp along this rugged stretch of coastline.

How to get there

To reach the launch site exit Highway 1 at William R. Hearst Memorial State Beach in San Simeon. Enter the State Beach and park in the lower parking lot adjacent to the beach. Restrooms, picnic facilities, and telephones are provided. Fee.

To reach the landing site, exit Highway 1 at the northern end of Moonstone Beach Drive which is about five and one-half miles south of San Simeon. Park on the south side of the bridge at Leffingwell Landing. A public launch ramp provides access to the beach, and parking is permitted along Moonstone Drive. No fee.

Camping

Tent and RV campsites are available at San Simeon State Park on Highway 1 about six miles southeast of William R. Hearst Memorial State Beach. For camping reservations, call ParkNet (800) 444-7275.

Hazards

Once outside the shelter of San Simeon Point, conditions can change dramatically. Unobstructed northwesterly winds blow onshore between Little Pico Creek and Leffingwell Landing. Waves can be large and conditions extremely choppy during the afternoon. Fog is common year-round. Plan an

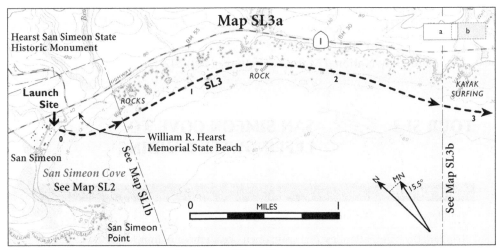

Tour SL3: San Simeon Cove to Leffingwell Landing

early start to allow ample time to reach Leffingwell Landing before the after-noon wind begins to blow.

Public access

Highway 1 parallels the coast, providing several pullouts and vista points for public access to the beaches. San Simeon State Beach extends from San Simeon Creek to Leffingwell Landing and is accessible to the public. This tour is within the Monterey Bay National Marine Sanctuary.

Kayak surfing

Good waves for kayak surfing can be found at Pico Creek.

Launching

Launch from the beach just west of the pier at William R. Hearst Memorial State Beach. Conditions are usually calm but a surf launching may be neces-sary.

Tour description

Pass the San Simeon Pier and head southeast toward the town of Cambria. The shoreline consists of sandy beaches separated by rocky headlands and offshore rocks of the Franciscan Formation.

The bluff along this section of coastline is steep. There are numerous sand beaches but large waves make landing difficult. Offshore there are several exposed rocks and shallow reefs. Kelp beds are sporadic, mostly appearing off the rocky headlands. Sea otters, sea lions, and harbor seals are commonly seen in the kelp beds. During the spring, on their leisurely northern migration, cow

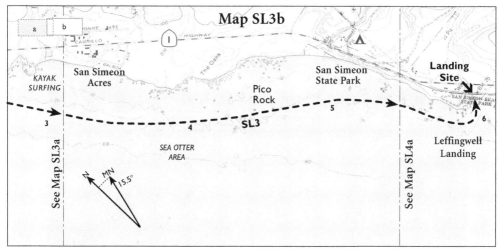

Tour SL3 (continued)

and calf gray-whale pairs stop in the kelp beds to rest and relax. At times, during calm weather, the whales lie motionless for an hour or more. The gray-whale calf is 15 to 18 feet long and weighs about 2500 pounds. The calf will gain an average of 180 pounds a day from the rich yogurt like milk produced from the mother. A full grown gray whale is about 40 feet long and weighs up to 45 tones. Fishing and scuba diving are great in the kelp beds off Pico Creek, San Simeon Creek and Leffingwell landing.

Landing

Leffingwell Landing is located on the south side of Leffingwell Point. Stay well offshore to avoid the shallow reef as you round the point. The waves in the cove are usually small and break close to the beach. A surf landing is rarely necessary. A concrete ramp, that extends from the road to the beach, provides easy access.

What to do afterward

The village of Cambria offers lodging, entertainment, fine dining, unique shops, and art galleries.

Alternate tour: SL2

For more information

William R. Hearst Memorial State Beach (805) 927-2068
Cambria Chamber of Commerce (805) 927-3624
US Coast Guard (805) 772-2167
Monterey Bay National Marine Sanctuary (408) 647-4201

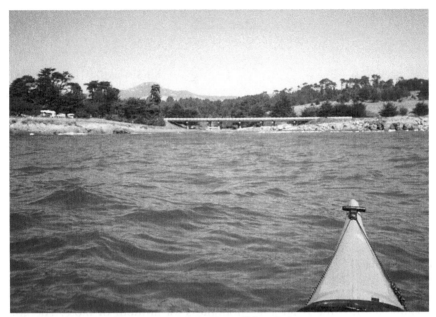

Avoid the shallow reef as you approach Leffingwell Landing

TOUR SL4 SHAMMEL PARK TO CAYUCOS PIER

Tour Details

Skill level:	Advanced
Trip length/type:	17.2 miles; one-way; open-ocean; six to seven hours
Chart/map:	NOAA Chart #s 18700 and 18703; USGS *Cambria* and *Cayucos* 7.5 min series

Summary

If a solitary kayak adventure on a remote section of coastline sounds like fun, this is the tour for you.

How to get there

To reach the launch site, exit Highway 1 at Windsor Boulevard (at the west end of Cambria) and proceed south about one-quarter mile to Shammel County Park. Park in the parking area on the south side of the park adjacent to the beach. Restrooms, picnic facilities, and telephones are available. No fee.

To reach the landing site, exit Highway 1 at Cayucos Drive in Cayucos (about 13 miles south of Cambria). Go south on Cayucos Drive for one-half mile and park in the parking lot on the west side of the pier. Restrooms and telephones are available at the Cayucos Pier. No fee.

Camping

Tent and RV campsites are available at San Simeon State Park approximately three miles north of Cambria on Highway 1. For camping reservations, call ParkNet (800) 444-7275.

Hazards

During large surf conditions there are few sheltered landing spots between Shammel Park and Estero Point. Watch for breaking water on offshore shoals. Southeast of Estero Point there are several protected landing spots, but the ocean-front property is privately owned. Don't plan on being able to drive your car down to the water to pick up your boat if you need to make an emergency landing. Get an early start to allow ample time to round Estero Point before the afternoon winds begin. Don't attempt this tour if weather reports call for strong northwesterly winds or high seas.

Public access

The shoreline is privately owned along this entire length of coastline.

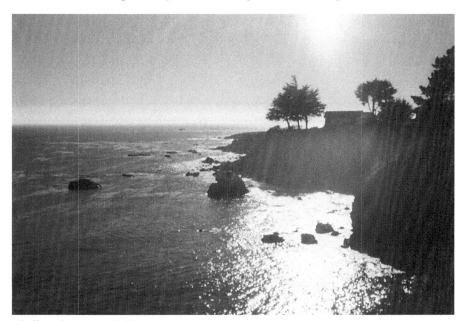

Bluffs at the west end of Cayucos

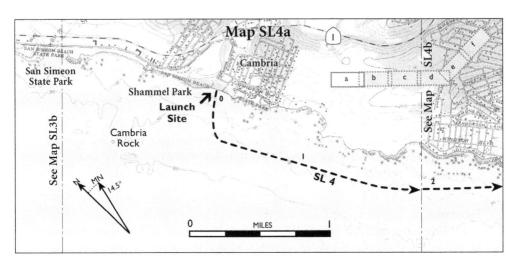

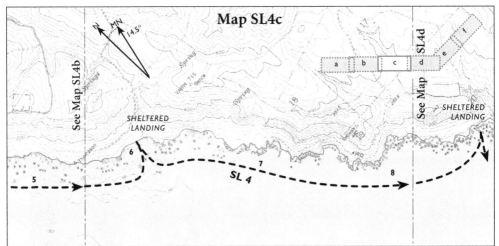

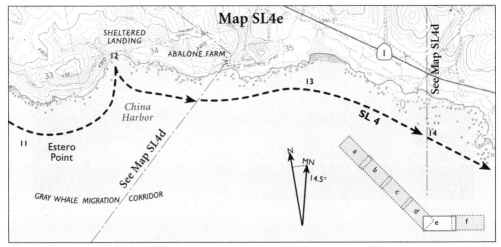

Tour SL4: Shammel Park to Cayucos Pier

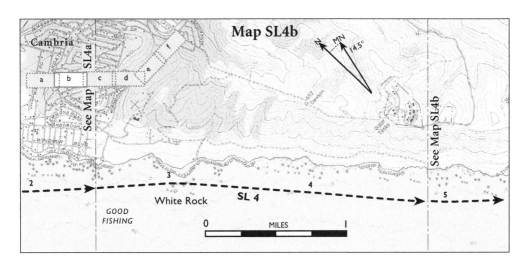

Map SL4b

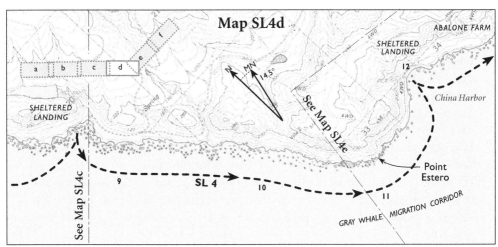

Map SL4d

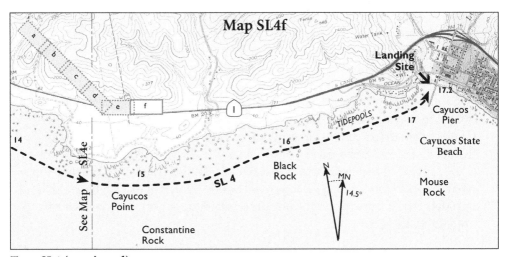

Map SL4f

Tour SL4 (continued)

Kayak surfing

The best waves for kayak surfing can be found at Cayucos Point, a local surf spot known as "Killers," about two miles west of Cayucos.

Launching

Launch from the sand beach adjacent to the parking lot at Shammel Park. The waves are powerful and break near the shore; there can be a strong undertow. Observe the conditions carefully before launching. A surf launch is frequently necessary.

Tour description

A shallow reef extends well offshore just south of the launch site. Watch carefully for sneaker waves before turning and heading south. Other than two isolated residences constructed within the last few years, the coastline between Cambria and Estero Point is totally undeveloped. The hills are gently rolling and grassy. Trees are sparse, beyond the Monterey-pine forests of Cambria. The marine terrace is narrow and the bluff is relatively low-lying and linear with few major headlands or sheltered embayments. Fishing is good in the kelp beds off White Rock. During relatively calm conditions, sheltered landings can be found at six and eight and three-quarters miles. There is an old fisherman's shack on the bluff overlooking the cove at eight and three-quarters miles. If you decide to go ashore, stay on the beach; the bluff-top property is all privately owned. Because this section of coast is so remote, you never know what you may stumble across on shore. Beach combing is an adventure and the tide pools are pristine. Harbor seals haul-out on many of the offshore rocks and sea otters are abundant. During the winter and spring, Estero point is a good location for viewing California gray whales.

At Estero Point the coastline turns east. China Harbor, in the lee of Estero Point, is sheltered from the northwest wind and swells and is an ideal spot for a lunch break. On the bluff (just to the east of China Harbor) is a commercial abalone farm, where abalone are grown in saltwater pools. Due to overfishing and disease, the natural abalone population in California has decreased significantly over the past 20 years.

Cayucos Point, about two miles west of the town of Cayucos, has good conditions for kayak surfing. The waves are powerful, however, and only experienced kayak surfers should attempt riding them. The local surfers have named the spot "Killers" for a good reason. Between Cayucos Point and Cayucos Creek, a shallow reef extends a long distance offshore. At low tide much of the reef is exposed, revealing a vast network of tide pools. Several sheltered landing spots offer easy access to the tide pools. Offshore, harbor seals and sea otter are commonly seen.

Landing

Land on the sand beach west of the Cayucos Pier. Conditions are frequently calm, but a surf landing may be necessary.

What to do afterward

You will probably be totally starved by the time you reach Cayucos. Fortunately there are several good restaurants within easy walking distance of the pier. The town of Cayucos is noted for its old town charm, beautiful beaches, and great weather.

Alternate tour: SL5

For more information

San Luis Obispo County Parks (805) 781-5219
Cayucos Chamber of Commerce (805) 995-1200
US Coast Guard (805) 772-2167

TOUR SL5 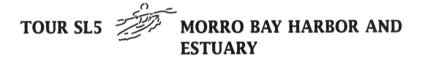 MORRO BAY HARBOR AND ESTUARY

Tour Details	
Skill level:	Beginner
Trip length/type:	11.3 miles; round-trip; bay; three to five hours (depending on the hiking time)
Chart/map:	NOAA Chart # 18703; USGS *Morro Bay South* 7.5 min series

Summary

This tour offers magnificent views of Morro Rock; some of the best kayak surfing in the state; a hike across the sand spit; and a meander through the quiet tidal channels and salt marshes of the Morro Bay Estuary.

How to get there

To reach the launch site exit Highway 1 about one-half mile east of Morro Bay at South Bay Boulevard. Proceed south on South Bay Boulevard for about a mile to State Park Road. Go right on State Park Road and follow the signs to Morro Bay State Park. Park across the street from the state park in the State Park Marina parking lot (behind the Bayside Cafe). Parking, restrooms, and telephones are available. No fee.

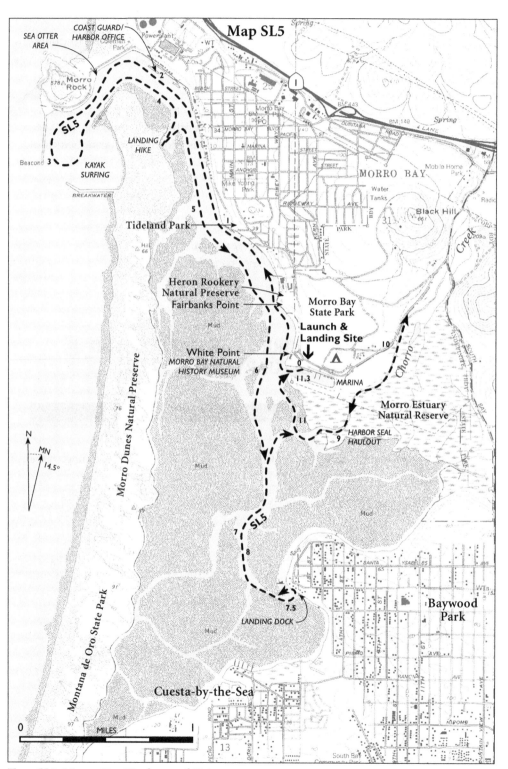

Tour SL5: Morro Bay Harbor and Estuary

Camping

Tent and RV campsites are available at Morro Bay State Park. For camping reservations, call ParkNet (800) 444-7275.

Hazards

Boat traffic can be congested; always follow the rules of the road. Be careful when approaching the harbor mouth. During the winter months, large waves break across the harbor entrance. If possible plan your trip route to have a following tidal current, so you will be exploring the estuary or shallow-water areas during a high tide.

Public access

Most of the shoreline in the harbor and estuary are public.

Kayak surfing

Some of the best kayak surfing in California can be found during the winter months inside the mouth to Morro Bay Harbor. The best conditions occur during low tide. Extreme caution must be exercised when riding these waves; the currents are strong and the waves can be very powerful. It's a good idea to check with the Harbor Patrol first.

Launching

Launch at the west end of the State Park Marina parking lot, adjacent to the rental-boat dock. There is no surf but the mud can be slippery.

Tour description

From the marina, head north toward Morro Rock. To the right, on the bluff overlooking the marina, is the Morro Bay Museum of Natural History. Across the bay is the sand spit and beyond is the open ocean. To the north of the Natural History Museum in the cluster of eucalyptus trees along the shoreline is the Morro Bay Blue Heron Rookery. Standing four feet tall with a wingspan of about six feet, the great blue heron is the largest of all the long-legged birds seen on the central coast of California. At low tide, the peak feeding time, herons can be seen standing motionless in the shallow water watching for small fish. During non-breeding seasons, the Morro Bay estuary may support as many as fifty blue herons. Other species commonly seen in the rookery are the white egret and the cormorant. North of the rookery is Tideland Park, a pleasant rest-stop with picnic facilities and restrooms.

From Tideland Park continue northward along the main channel toward Morro Rock. On your right is the Embarcadero, home of the fishing fleet, the US Coast Guard, and the Morro Bay Harbor Patrol. At the Pacific Gas and Electric power plant the main channel turns left toward Morro Rock. Morro

Rock is one of the "Seven Sisters," a linear series of volcanic peaks extending from Morro Bay to San Luis Obispo. The volcanic intrusions occurred about 22 to 24 million years ago and probably never reached the surface to form true volcanoes. The soft sediment and ash that once covered the intrusion at Morro Rock have eroded leaving the 581-foot high rock we see today. The rock was named "El Moro" by the Spanish explorer Juan Rodriguez Cabrillo in 1542. At the time of Cabrillo's visit, Morro Rock was an offshore island with channels leading to the bay on both sides. In 1933, a causeway was constructed closing the north channel and connecting the rock to the mainland. In 1969, Morro Rock was established as an ecological reserve.

Morro Bay harbor entrance, one of the roughest on the west coast, is closed to boat traffic for up to 40 days a year because of rough seas. Nearly every winter, lives are lost when careless boaters try to enter the harbor during storm conditions. Never risk crossing the harbor mouth if waves are breaking in the entrance channel. If you are experienced at kayak surfing, you may want to sample some of the waves that break just inside the harbor entrance. At low tide, large swells roll across the shallow water creating the perfect wave for a kayak. It can be an experience you won't soon forget. Unless you are an experienced kayaker, stay clear of the harbor mouth during stormy conditions.

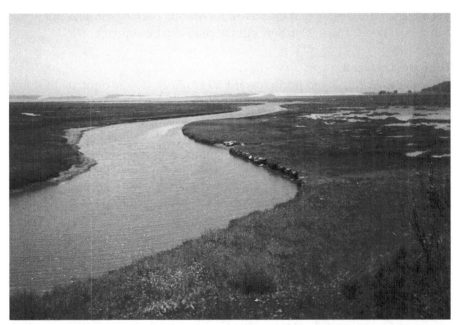

Morro Bay Estuary consists of 2300 acres of mud flats, eel grass, tidal wetlands, and open-water channels

Back in the harbor, paddle south along the inside of the sand spit. Land your kayak and walk across the sand spit. It's a good idea to wear shoes or your wet-suit boots and bring an extra jacket in case it gets cold. On the seaward side of the sand spit is a beautiful, wide, sand beach great for beach combing. Driftwood, sand dollars, and seashells are abundant. Large piles (middens) of shells and bones, left by the Chumash Indians can still be seen. Swimming is not advised due to the powerful waves and strong undertows— not to mention the frigid water.

From the sand spit, follow the main channel back to the State Park Marina from which you began. You can end the tour at this point or continue into the Morro Bay Estuary. The estuary consists of 2300 acres of mud flats, eel grass, tidal wetlands, and open water channels. Tidal channels meander through the wetlands, offering a closeup view of the wildlife. Over two dozen threatened and endangered species live in the watershed, including: peregrine falcon, brown pelican, sea otter, black rail, snowy plover, steelhead trout, salt marsh bird's beak, and Morro manzanita. At high tide it is possible to paddle a short distance up Chorro Creek, which is one of several freshwater creeks feeding the estuary. Check your tide tables to avoid getting stuck in the mud flats on an outgoing tide. Baywood Park, a quaint waterfront village at the southern end of the estuary, has a landing dock, shops and restaurants.

Return to the State Park Marina.

Landing

Land at the State Park Marina where you launched.

What to do afterward

The Bayside Cafe, located at the Marina, has very good food. Service is great and prices are reasonable. The Natural History Museum, is on the promontory overlooking the Marina. The Morro Bay Golf Course is nearby and Morro Bay State Park is across State Park Road from the marina. The city of Morro Bay has a wonderful downtown with a variety of shops and fine restaurants. At Christmas time, Morro Bay has a spectacular lighted boat parade. Get some lights for your kayak and plan on entering the parade.

Alternate tour: LR2

For more information

US Coast Guard (805) 772-2167
Morro Bay Harbor Department (805) 772-6254
Marine Weather (805) 772-4620

TOUR SL6 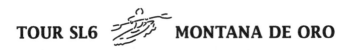 MONTANA DE ORO

Tour Details

Skill level:	Advanced (can be suitable for intermediate level during calm conditions)
Trip length/type:	4.1 miles; round-trip; open-ocean; two to three hours
Chart/map:	NOAA Chart #s 18703 and 18704; USGS *Morro Bay South* 7.5 min series

Summary

For a different perspective than most visitors get of Montana de Oro State Park, try this short but action-packed adventure. Sea caves, natural arches, rich kelp beds, and abundant wildlife will all be yours to experience if you can just get the weather to cooperate.

How to get there

To reach the launch site exit Highway 101 at Los Osos Valley Road and proceed 12 miles west to Montana de Oro State Park. Park in the parking lot at Spooner's Cove. Restrooms, picnic facilities, and telephones are available. No fee.

Camping

Tent and RV campsites are available at Montana de Oro State Park. For camping reservations, call ParkNet (800) 444-7275.

Hazards

Conditions are very unpredictable and should be assessed carefully before launching. Don't count on many sheltered landing spots along this route if there is a strong swell. Conditions are often choppy and unsettled in Spooner's Cove due to waves reflected off the vertical bluffs.

Public access

The shoreline north of Coon Creek is accessible to the public.

Kayak surfing

The shoreline is rocky and the waves are powerful and generally not suitable for kayak surfing.

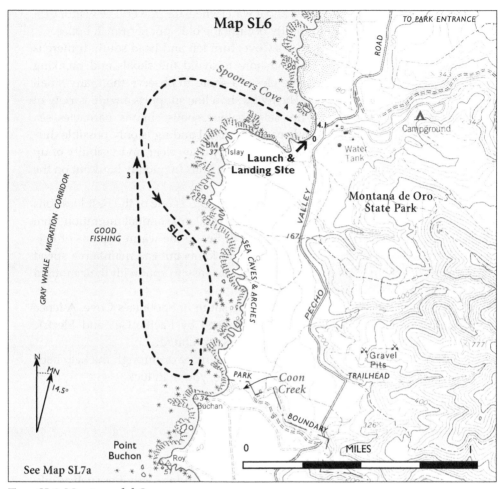

Tour SL6: Montana del Oro

Launching

Launch from the sand beach adjacent to the parking lot at Spooner's Cove. The waves are usually small and break close to shore but a surf launch may be necessary.

Tour description

In the late 1800s, coastal steamers stopped in Spooner's Cove to load and unload supplies for the Spooner family, early ranchers in the area. On the south bluff overlooking the cove, a warehouse was built with a long wooden chute to deliver goods to the waiting ships. The remains of the warehouse and wharf can still be seen. The Spooners built a ranch house, a complex of barns, a creamery, stables, sheds, and a waterwheel for power. The visitor center and park headquarters currently occupy the old Spooner ranch house.

After paddling out of Spooner's Cove, turn left and head south. If there is a swell, paddle a safe distance offshore to avoid the shoals and breaking waves. If the sea is calm, paddle close to shore to observe the many small islets, reefs, arches, and caves. The rocky shoreline supports a wide variety of plants and animals including mussels, abalone, snails, chitons, barnacles, sea stars, hermit crabs, urchins, and sea anenomes. Landing is only possible during very calm conditions. The water is usually quite clear, and visibility of up to 40 feet is not unusual. Harbor seals and sea lions frequently haul-out on the offshore rocks and islets.

During the winter and spring, Montana de Oro is one of the best locations for viewing the California gray whale on its 5000 mile annual migration from their summer feeding grounds in the Arctic Sea to the warm lagoons of Baja California. Gray whales cruise at about four knots but can maintain a speed of ten knots for up to an hour. The whales are easy to spot with their mottled gray color and barnacle covered back.

Coon Creek is about a two mile paddle south of Spooner's Cove. A fence separates the state park from property owned by Pacific Gas and Electric Company. Trespassing on PG&E property is prohibited.

Return to Spooner's Cove via the shoreline route or through the kelp beds further offshore. If you brought a fishing pole, you're in luck.

Landing
Land at Spooner's Cove where you launched.

What to do afterward
Montana de Oro State Park offers a variety of outdoor activities such as hiking, biking, horseback riding, and surfing. There are picnic facilities, self-guiding nature trails, and a visitor center with information and nature displays.

Alternate tour: SL5

For more information
Morro Bay Harbor Department (805) 772-6254
Montana de Oro Ranger Headquarters (805) 528-0513

TOUR SL7 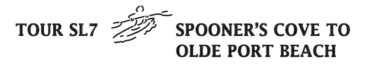 SPOONER'S COVE TO OLDE PORT BEACH

Tour Details	
Skill level:	Advanced
Trip length:	17.0 miles; one way; open-ocean; six to seven hours
Chart/map:	NOAA Chart #s 18703 and 18704; *USGS Morro Bay South, Port San Luis,* and *Pismo Beach* 7.5 min series

Summary

Little has changed since the Chumash Indians inhabited this remote section of unspoiled coastline. During winter and spring this trip offers one of the best opportunities for viewing California gray whales on their annual migration.

How to get there

To reach the launch site exit Highway 101 at Los Osos Valley Road and proceed 12 miles west to Montana de Oro State Park. Park in the parking lot at Spooner's Cove. Restrooms, picnic facilities, and telephones are available. No fee.

To reach the landing site, exit Highway 101 at Avila Beach Road and proceed west four miles to the Olde Port Beach boat launch. Park on Avila Beach Drive. Restrooms and telephones are available. No fee.

Camping

Tent and RV campsites are available at Montana de Oro State Park. For camping reservations, call ParkNet (800) 444-7275.

Hazards

Conditions are very unpredictable and should be assessed carefully before launching. Don't count on many sheltered landing spots along the route if there is a strong swell. Conditions are often choppy and unsettled in Spooner's Cove due to waves reflected off the vertical bluffs. Give all headlands plenty of room during high seas. Winds are usually strongest north of Diablo Canyon, so get an early start. Boat traffic in Port San Luis can be congested; always follow the rules of the road.

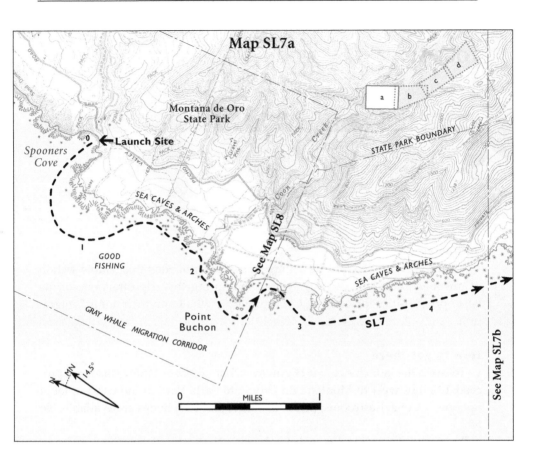

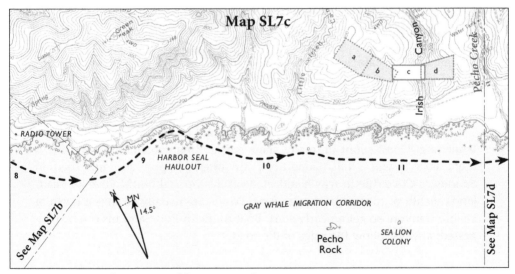

Tour SL7: Spooner's Cove to Olde Port Beach

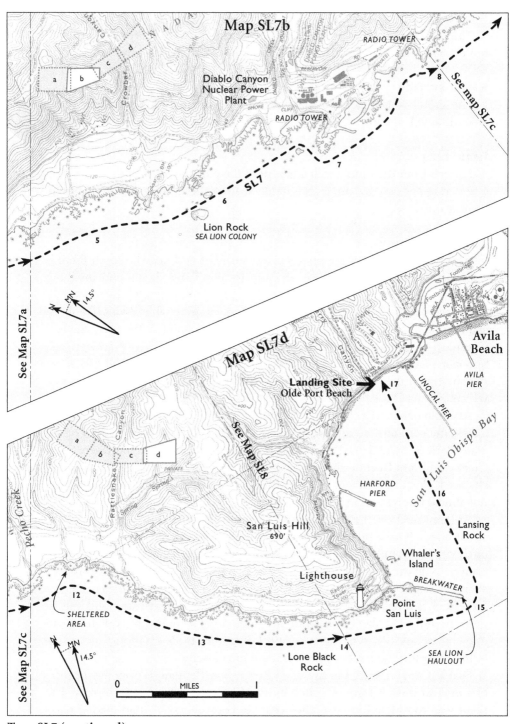

Map SL7b

RADIO TOWER

Diablo Canyon
Nuclear Power
Plant

RADIO TOWER

See map SL7c

8

7

SL7

6

5

Lion Rock
SEA LION COLONY

See Map SL7a

a b c d

See Map SL7c

N MN 14.5°

Map SL7d

See Map SL8

Avila
Beach

*AVILA
PIER*

Landing Site ➤
Olde Port Beach

17

UNOCAL PIER

San Luis Obispo Bay

a b c d

PRIVATE

Pecho Creek

Rattlesnake Canyon

Spring

Spring

San Luis Hill
690'

HARFORD
PIER

16

Lansing
Rock

Whaler's
Island

Lighthouse

BREAKWATER

Point
San Luis

15

12

SHELTERED
AREA

13

14

Lone Black
Rock

SEA LION
HAULOUT

See Map SL7c

N MN 14.5°

0   MILES   1

Tour SL7 (continued)

Public access

The beach north of Coon Creek is accessible to the public. From Coon Creek to Port San Luis, is owned by Pacific Gas and Electric Company.

Kayak surfing

The shoreline is rocky and the waves are powerful and generally not suitable for kayak surfing.

Launching

Launch from the sand beach adjacent to the parking lot at Spooner's Cove. The waves are usually small and break close to shore but a surf launch may be necessary.

Tour description

After paddling out of Spooner's Cove, turn left and head south. If there is a swell, paddle a safe distance offshore to avoid the shoals and breaking waves.

As you paddle along this pristine coastline, imagine what it was like thousands of years ago when the Chumash Indians inhabited the area. Several Chumash villages dating back 9000 years have been discovered between Spooner's Cove and Port San Luis. The Chumash were hunters and gatherers, depending on the sea for much of their food. The *tomol*, a wood plank canoe which they used for fishing, was made by hand from planks of driftwood.

At about one land mile south of Spooner's Cove (two miles paddle) is Coon Creek, the southern boundary of the State Park. The land to the south of the State Park is owned by Pacific Gas and Electric Company. Between Coon Creek and Point Buchon there are hundreds of sea caves of various sizes and shapes. Colorful green and red algae grow on the moist cavern walls appearing almost fluorescent in the dim light.

At Point Buchon, the coastline turns southeast. There is a red whistle buoy about one-half mile offshore. The gray whale migration corridor passes close offshore. Three miles south of Point Buchon are Lion Rock and the Diablo Canyon Nuclear Power Plant. The large rock lies about one-quarter mile offshore. Passage between Lion Rock and the mainland is possible on a calm day. Lion Rock is inhabited by hundreds of sea lions that always seem anxious to greet friendly kayakers. On land, sea lions appear awkward, but they can often move faster than humans for short distances. Bulls are highly protective of their territory, so never approach them too closely.

Diablo Canyon, once the site of a Chumash settlement, is now the location of a nuclear power plant operated by Pacific Gas and Electric Company. The plant was completed in 1986 after years of controversy. A man-made breakwater has been constructed to protect the plant facilities. Three miles south of

Diablo Canyon is Pecho Rock, a large offshore rock used by sea lions as a haul-out. There are three partially submerged rocks on the south side of Pecho Rock. Passage is possible between the mainland and the rocks but watch for shoaling waves. The rocks can be difficult to spot during white-capping conditions.

From Pecho Rock to the Point San Luis Lighthouse is about five miles. The Victorian-style lighthouse constructed on Point San Luis was completed in 1890. Originally named the Port Harford Light, it is one of seven West Coast lighthouses of similar design. The original Fresnel lens was shipped separately from France on four different vessels so the entire lens would not be lost if one of the ships sank. In the late 1800s Port Harford was a thriving whaling station. Whaling facilities were located on Whaler's Island and Smith Island. Whale oil was used to fuel the original light until replaced by electricity. Today the light is automated.

From the Point San Luis Lighthouse, proceed around the end of the breakwater. Pass seaward of the rocky shoal near the tip of the breakwater. Sea lions frequently haul-out at the end of the breakwater. Follow the channel-marker buoys to the Harford Pier. The Olde Port Beach launch ramp is located about one-quarter mile west of the Unocal Pier.

Landing

Land on the beach in front of the launch ramp at Olde Port Beach. The waves are usually small and break near the shore at Olde Port Beach, but a surf landing is sometimes necessary. Be sure to stay clear of designated swimming areas, which are identified by white buoys. Avoid driving on the beach; it's easy to get stuck in the soft sand.

What to do afterward

By the time you have completed this marathon paddle, you may not have the energy to do anything but sleep. Fat Cats Restaurant at Port San Luis and the Olde Port Inn at the end of the Harford Pier both have good seafood and the prices are reasonable.

Alternate tour: SL5

For more information

Montana de Oro Ranger Headquarters (805) 528-0513
Port San Luis Harbor District Office (805) 595-5400

TOUR SL8 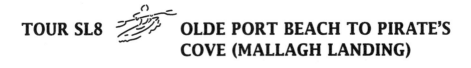 OLDE PORT BEACH TO PIRATE'S COVE (MALLAGH LANDING)

Tour Details

Skill level:	Beginner
Trip length/type:	9.3 miles; round trip; bay; three to four hours
Chart/map:	NOAA Chart # 18704; USGS *Port San Luis* and *Pismo Beach* 7.5 min series

Summary

Explore bustling Port San Luis, the tranquility of the San Luis Obispo Creek estuary, and the spectacular setting of Pirate's Cove on this relatively easy trip perfect for beginners.

How to get there

To reach the launch site, exit Highway 101 at Avila Beach Road and proceed west four miles to the Olde Port Beach boat launch. Park on Avila Beach Road. Restrooms and telephones are available. No fee.

Camping

Tent and RV campsites are available at Pismo State Beach, on Highway 1 eight miles south of Avila Beach. For camping reservations, call ParkNet (800) 444-7275. Camping is also available at Avila Hot Springs Spa and Resort in Avila Beach. For reservations call (805) 595-2359.

Hazards

This section of coastline has a southern exposure and is partly sheltered from northwesterly winds and swells.Watch carefully for shallow, submerged rocks in the Pirate's Cove area. Conditions are usually calm in the morning, with a light to moderate offshore breeze in the afternoon. Fog occurs occasionally, but burn-off is usually early. Boat traffic can be congested; always follow the rules of the road.

Public access

Most of the shoreline is public with the exception of the Unocal property between Avila Beach and Pirate's Cove.

Kayak surfing

The waves are small and not suitable for kayak surfing.

Launching

Launch from the beach in front of the launch ramp at Olde Port Beach. The waves are usually small and break near the shore at Olde Port Beach, but a surf landing is sometimes necessary. Be sure to stay clear of designated swimming areas, which are identified by white buoys. Avoid driving on the beach; it's easy to get stuck in the soft sand.

Tour description

From the Olde Port Beach boat launch, head southwest toward the Harford Pier. The Harford Pier was built in 1873 by John Harford to service steamships carrying passengers and freight up and down the California coast. A steam railroad connected the city of San Luis Obispo and the port. After the completion of the Southern Pacific Railroad through San Luis Obispo in 1890, activity at the port declined, and in 1941, service on the steam railroad was discontinued. Today Port San Luis supports an active commercial and sport-fishing fleet. Facilities on the pier include fish markets, a tackle shop, and a restaurant. The harbor bustles with activity as crab, rock fish, halibut, and albacore (when in season) are unloaded from the waiting boats and processed for shipping. Watching the busy harbor from a kayak can be very exciting. Beneath the pier, hungry sea lions wait for a handout, while overhead, seagulls and pelicans circle in anticipation. The brown pelican circles at a height of 20-40 feet above the water looking for its prey, then dives straight into the

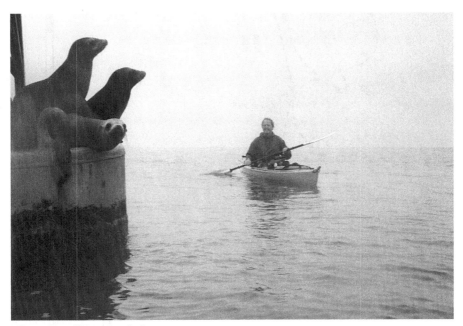

The author off Port San Luis

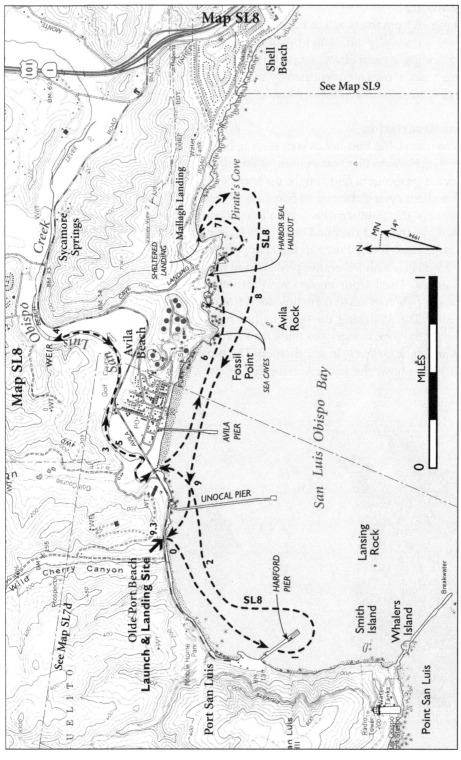

Tour SL8 Olde Port Beach to Pirate's Cove (Mallagh Landing)

water, making a huge splash. After catching the fish, the pelican returns to the surface to drain its pouch and swallow its catch. Paddle beneath the pier and look up. The dining room tables in the Olde Port Inn restaurant have glass table-tops so diners can view the water beneath the pier. It's fun to watch the looks on the diner's faces as you pass beneath their fish and chips.

From the Harford Pier head back past Olde Port Beach and continue past the Unocal Pier. On your left, just past the Unocal Pier, is the mouth of San Luis Obispo Creek. If conditions are calm (as they usually are), land on the beach next to the bridge and portage your kayak to the estuary. During most of the year it is possible to paddle about a mile upstream. There are many birds and the still water of the estuary offers a nice change from the restless ocean. Watch out for flying golf balls; the San Luis Bay Golf Course surrounds the estuary.

Back on the bay, resume paddling east past the Avila Pier. Stay to seaward of the white buoys marking the swimming areas. Fossil Point, the rocky head-land at the east end of the beach, is notched with sea caves. Some of the caves are high on the cliff, well above current sea level, indicating a relatively rapid rate of geologic uplift in the area.

About one-half mile east of Fossil Point is Pirate's Cove. The kelp beds in this area are very thick and can make paddling difficult. Pirate's Cove is a clothing-optional beach. Landing is easy and the weather is almost always sunny and warm. The Padres from Mission San Luis Obispo used this natural rock landing to transfer hides prepared at the Mission onto waiting ships. In 1860, a warehouse was built on the bluff top and a chute was constructed to facilitate loading of goods. You can still see a rock stairway and the large steel rings embedded in the rock where ships were tied. From Pirate's Cove, return to Olde Port Beach.

Landing

Land at Olde Port Beach where you launched.

What to do afterward

For a massage and a warm mineral bath, Sycamore Mineral Springs is located on Avila Beach Road one mile west of Highway 101.

Alternate tour: LR3

For more information

Port San Luis Harbor District Office (805) 595-5400

TOUR SL9 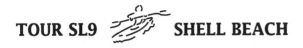 SHELL BEACH

Tour Details

Skill level:	Beginner
Trip length/type:	4.4 miles; round-trip; open-ocean/sheltered; two to three hours
Chart/map:	NOAA Chart #s 18700 and 18704; USGS *Pismo Beach* 7.5 min series

Summary

Explore the sea caves and meander through the offshore rocks which are home to harbor seals, pelicans, cormorants, and gulls. This idyllic setting is the perfect sunset cruise.

How to get there

To reach the launch site, exit Highway 101 at Spyglass Drive in Shell Beach. Proceed one mile southeast on Shell Beach Road. Turn right on Vista del Mar Avenue. Park on the street at the corner of Vista del Mar Avenue and Ocean Boulevard. Street parking and picnic facilities are available. No fee.

Camping

Tent and RV campsites are available at Pismo State Beach, on Highway 1 two miles south of Shell Beach. For camping reservations, call ParkNet (800) 444-7275.

Hazards

This section of coastline has a southwest exposure and is partly sheltered from the northwesterly winds and swells. Watch carefully for shallow, submerged rocks. Conditions are usually calm in the morning, with a light to moderate side-shore breeze in the afternoon. Fog occurs occasionally but burn-off is usually early. Wear a helmet and PFD, and carry a waterproof flashlight when exploring the caves.

Public access

Most of the shoreline is privately owned. Ocean Park (located between Vista del Mar Avenue and and Capistrano Avenue) and Margo Dodd Park are public.

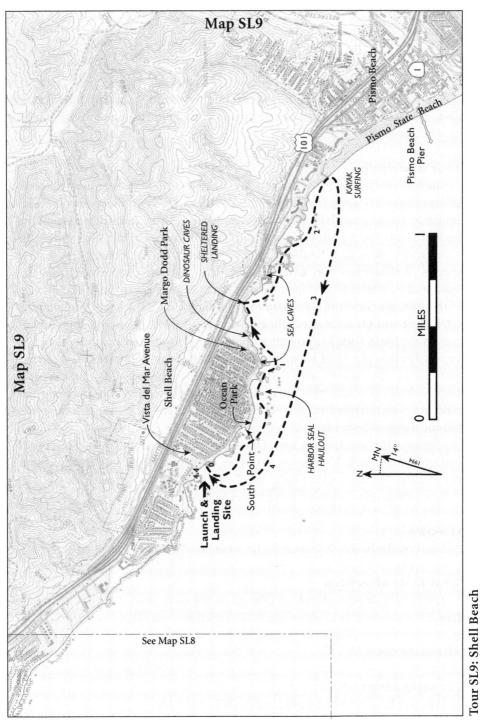

Map SL9

Map SL9

Pismo Beach

Pismo State Beach

Pismo Beach Pier

KAYAK SURFING

SHELTERED LANDING

DINOSAUR CAVES

Margo Dodd Park

SEA CAVES

Vista del Mar Avenue

Shell Beach

Ocean Park

HARBOR SEAL HAULOUT

South Point

Launch & Landing Site

MILES

See Map SL8

Tour SL9: Shell Beach

Kayak surfing

The waves at Pismo Beach, at the southeast end of this tour, are good for kayak surfing.

Launching

Launch from the beach at the foot of the stairway at Vista del Mar Avenue. Conditions are usually calm except during winter storms when a surf launch may be necessary.

Tour description

Shallow reefs border the launch site at Vista del Mar Avenue. The reefs extend about 100 yards from the beach. Paddle out beyond the reefs then head southeast toward South Point. A large residence with a windmill stands on the bluff at South Point. Paddle close to shore if conditions permit. Numerous off-shore rocks serve as a haul-out for harbor seals and a rookery for several species of shorebirds. Off Margo Dodd Park is an islet separated from the mainland by a narrow channel. A large sea cave extends through the middle of the islet, and on calm days you can paddle through the cave. The water is often clear and ideal for snorkeling. Just beyond the islet are two large openings in the bluff. Paddle into either opening and land your boat on the beach inside. There is plenty of room for several boats. Several hundred feet farther east are the "Dinosaur Caves." This extensive labyrinth got its name from a large concrete dinosaur that once stood on top of the bluff. I understand the dinosaur was intended to be a tourist attraction. The dinosaur is long gone, but the name still stands.

Continue to the southeast from Dinosaur Caves about one mile to the north end of Pismo Beach. Numerous sea caves are found along this entire section of coastline. The waves off Pismo Beach can be good for kayak surfing.

From Pismo Beach return to Vista del Mar Avenue.

Landing

Land on the beach at Vista del Mar Avenue where you launched.

What to do afterward

The historic Mission San Luis Obispo de Tolosa is located in the city of San Luis Obispo which is 12 miles north of Shell Beach on Highway 101.

Alternate tour: LR3

For more information

Port San Luis Harbor District Office (805) 595-5400

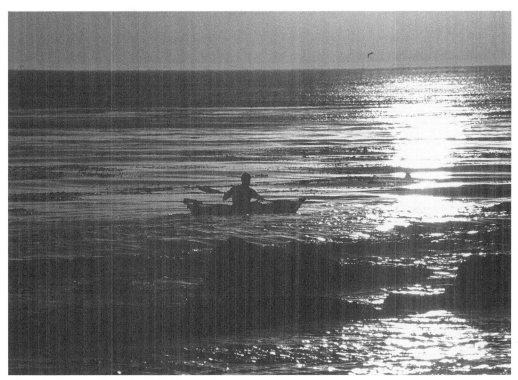

Shell Beach, San Luis Obispo County

Santa Barbara County Tours

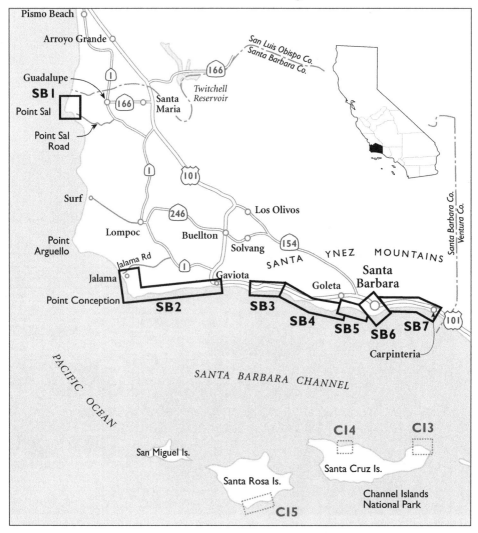

Tour		Skill Level	Length
SB1:	Point Sal Beach to Mussel Point	Advanced	8.5 miles
SB2:	Jalama Beach Park to Gaviota Beach State Park	Advanced	20.0 miles
SB3:	Refugio State Beach to El Capitan State Beach	Beginner	6.0 miles
SB4:	El Capitan State Beach to Goleta Beach Co. Park	Advanced	13.8 miles
SB5:	Goleta Beach to Arroyo Burro Beach County Park	Intermediate	5.4 miles
SB6:	Arroyo Burro Beach Co. Park to Santa Barbara Harbor		
		Beginner	5.0 miles
SB7:	Santa Barbara Harbor to Carpinteria Beach	Intermediate	11.0 miles

Chapter 4

Santa Barbara County

It was a gray morning and we were cold and wet. Our first attempt to launch through the surf had ended in a dumping. After bailing the cockpit and securing the deck gear that was swept off by the waves, we were finally on our way. The wind was light as we headed south toward Point Conception.

It had been an hour since we launched and we didn't seem any closer to our destination. Our arms were tiring and it felt as if we were paddling uphill. The seas were coming from behind us but the wind and a stiff current were coming from directly ahead. This unusual combination made the waves very steep and paddling difficult. Our tandem kayak was twenty feet long and seaworthy but we were still taking a lot of water over the bow.

As we finally neared the point we could see waves breaking on a reef nearly one-quarter mile offshore. A loud foghorn seemed to be sending an ominous warning so we headed a little further west to avoid the sharp rocks that could quickly put a hole through our thin fiberglass hull. About one-half mile southwest of the point, and finally clear of the reef, we turned east. Suddenly a large, cresting wave slammed into the side of our kayak, nearly throwing us into the sea. The steep waves that had been coming from astern were now hitting us broadside. We adjusted our course slightly to the north to gain some stability.

As we progressed eastward, into the lee of Point Conception, the seas began to calm. I breathed a sigh of relief as we rounded a low, rocky headland and entered a large sheltered bay. It was as if we had entered another world. The wind died and the sun was shining brightly. We headed for a sandy beach at the northeast corner of the bay.

After lunch and a brief reprieve from the morning's paddle, we were back on the water heading east. A vast expanse of glistening kelp extended far out to sea. We hugged the shoreline to avoid the kelp's tangled maze. A dry, warm breeze, scented with sage, blew gently off the land, and the towering peaks of the Santa Ynez Mountains seemed to shimmer in the warm summer sunlight. As we passed another low headland, the sea was like glass and the faint silhouettes of the Channel Islands seemed suspended on the endless horizon. The crystal blue water was transparent and the sparkling rays of sunshine danced across the sandy sea bottom. I took a deep breath and closed my eyes, capturing the moment forever.

— Point Conception, July 14, 1996

TOUR SB1 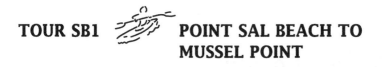 POINT SAL BEACH TO MUSSEL POINT

Tour Details

Skill level:	Advanced
Trip length/type:	8.5 miles; round-trip; open-ocean; three to four hours
Chart/map:	NOAA Chart #18700; USGS *Point Sal* 7.5 min series

Summary

If you are looking for that secret spot where none of your friends has ever paddled, and which no one has heard of, your search is over. It's unlikely you will see another person on this trip along one of the most remote sections of California coastline.

How to get there

To reach the launch site, exit Highway 1 south of the city of Guadalupe on Brown Road. Proceed west on Brown Road for about four miles to Point Sal Road. Turn right on Point Sal Road, and go about five miles west to Point Sal State Beach. The road is poorly maintained, partly unpaved, often impassable during winter storms, and may be temporarily closed during missile launches at Vandenberg Air Force Base. Parking is available. No fee.

Camping

Camping is permitted at Point Sal Beach. There are no facilities or fee.

Hazards

Shallow reefs extending seaward from both Point Sal and Mussel Rock should be avoided. Listen to the local weather forecast and don't bother making the drive to Point Sal if strong winds or high seas are forecast. Thick fog can occur at any time of the year and is very unpredictable.

Public access

Point Sal Beach, Paradise Beach, and the Guadalupe-Nipomo Dunes Preserve are accessible to the public.

Kayak surfing

Point Sal State Beach is noted for its good surf.

Launching

Launch from the beach in front of the parking lot at Point Sal State Beach. Kayaks must be carried from the parking lot down a steep dirt trail to the sand beach. A surf launch is usually necessary.

Tour description

From the launch site proceed north toward the rocky bluff at the end of the beach. The bluff should offer some protection from a northwesterly wind. In the late 1800s there was a small port at Point Sal. Goods produced in the Santa Maria Valley were shipped from a small wharf that stood on the beach near the bluff. Nothing remains of the original buildings or pier today.

From the north end of the beach, follow the rocky shoreline west toward Point Sal. The bubble-shaped rock outcropping along the shoreline is called pillow basalt. It was formed about 150 million years ago when molten magma, extruded from undersea volcanoes, was quickly cooled by the ocean water. The steeply sloping hillsides above the point are vegetated with grass and coastal sage. In the springtime, the slopes are brightened by the yellow flowers of the giant coreopsis, a plant similar to the sunflower. The coreopsis is a California native plant which is found only on the central California coast and the Channel Islands.

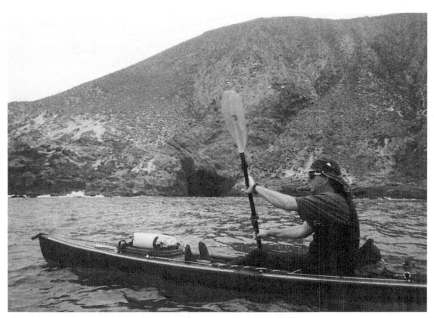

Sea cave on the south side of Point Sal

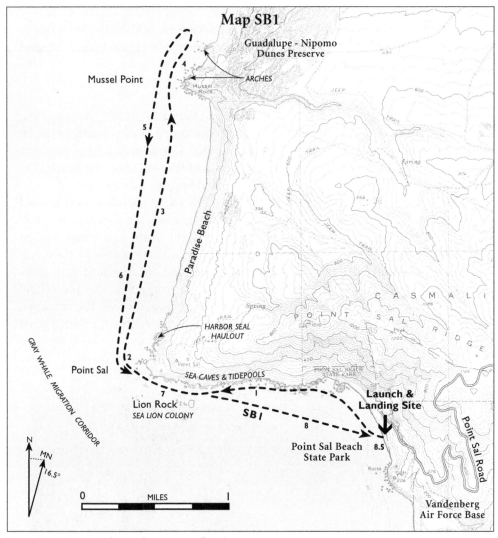

Tour SB1: Point Sal Beach to Mussel Point

Proceed cautiously when passing around Point Sal. Submerged offshore rocks with breaking waves and strong currents extend approximately one-half mile west of the point. Lion Rock, just south of the point, is a favorite haul-out for sea lions. Passage between Point Sal and Lion Rock can be hazardous during rough seas. During the late spring, cow and calf California gray whale pairs often stop to rest in the shelter of Point Sal on their northward migration. Sea caves and tide pools in the lee of the point can be explored during calm conditions.

From Point Sal proceed north. Mussel Point, which is approximately two miles north of Point Sal, should be clearly visible. The long, sandy beach between Mussel Point and Point Sal is known as Paradise Beach. If the waves are calm, a surf landing can be made at the north end of the beach in the shelter of Mussel Point.

Paradise Beach is seldom visited and is excellent for beach combing. Freshwater springs, supporting a variety of endemic plants, seep from the base of the cliff. At the north end of the beach a small waterfall cascades over the face of the bluff year-round. Several large rocks lie off Mussel Point. A natural rock arch connects one of the rocks to the point. Piles of discarded shells and bones, remnants of the Chumash Indians who inhabited the area for thousands of years, are scattered across the marine terrace. Farther up on the wind-blown slopes are mounds of flaked chert rock. Chert, because of its hardness and its conchoidal fracture, was used by the Chumash for a variety of tools and weapons including knives, scrapers, drills, and projectile points.

Mussel Point is within the Guadalupe-Nipomo Dunes Preserve. Mussel Rock Dune, which reaches a height of 500 feet, is the highest beach dune in the western United States. At least 18 species of rare plants and animals are found in the dunes. One of the last known nesting colonies of the endangered California least tern, a shorebird once common along the central and southern California coastline, is located in the preserve. Due to the strong winds and waves, landing on the north side of Mussel Point is not suggested. From Mussel Point, return to Point Sal Beach.

Landing
Land on the beach below the parking lot where you launched.

What to do afterward
A hiking trail leads from the north end of the Point Sal Beach to Point Sal. The trail is poorly maintained and not marked. The Guadalupe-Nipomo Dunes Preserve, an 18-mile stretch of coastal dunes with day-use hiking trails, is located at the end of Main Street, west of Guadalupe.

Alternate tour: SL8

For more information
Santa Barbara District Office, California State Parks (805) 899-1400
La Purisima Historical Monument (805) 733-3713

TOUR SB2 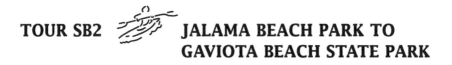 JALAMA BEACH PARK TO GAVIOTA BEACH STATE PARK

Tour Details	
Skill level:	Advanced
Trip length/type:	20.0 miles; one-way; open-ocean; seven to eight hours
Chart/map:	NOAA Chart #18721; USGS *Point Conception, Sacate* and *Gaviota* 7.5 min series

Summary

The mother of all California points, Point Conception is referred to by many as the "Cape Horn of the West Coast." This lengthy and difficult paddle, suitable for only the most advanced paddlers, is a captivating experience you won't soon forget.

How to get there

To reach the launch site, exit Highway 1 at Jalama Road and drive west about 15 miles to Jalama Beach Park. Parking, restrooms, picnic facilities, and telephones are available. Fee.

To reach the landing site, exit Highway 101 at Gaviota Beach State Park. Parking, restrooms, picnic facilities and telephones are available. Fee.

Camping

Camping is available at Jalama Beach Park. Individual campsites are available on a first-come/first-served basis. Reservations can be made for group camping. For group reservations call (805) 934-6211. Camping is also available at Gaviota Beach State Park. For camping reservations, call ParkNet (800) 444-7275.

Hazards

Conditions can be very unpredictable. The sea may be smooth and calm at Jalama and at the same time, rough and windy at Point Conception, which is only five miles away. This paddle should be attempted only during the most ideal conditions. Strong variable winds and currents can make the passage around Point Conception slow and tiring. The wind and waves frequently come from opposite directions, creating a very choppy and turbulent sea.

East of Point Conception, conditions are likely to be somewhat calmer. Winds often blow from the east in the morning, becoming northwesterly or

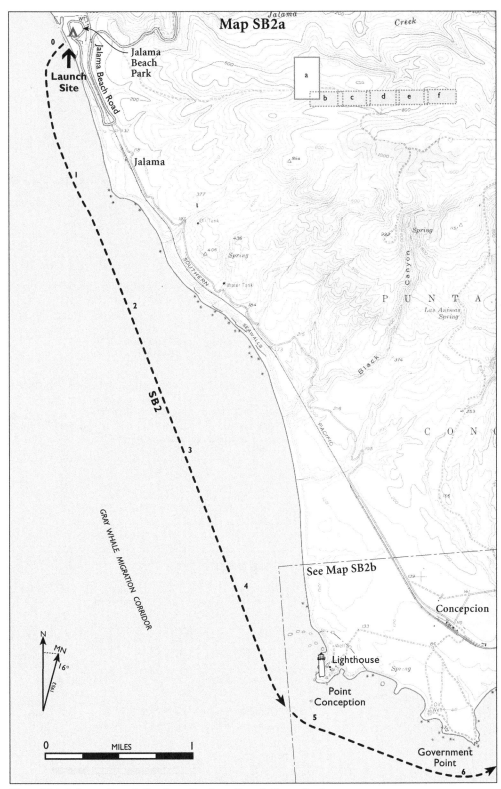

Map SB2a

Jalama Creek

Jalama Beach Park

Launch Site

Jalama Beach Road

Jalama

SOUTHERN

Oil Tank

Spring

Water Tank

SEA WALLS

PACIFIC

Black

Canyon

P U N T A

Las Animas Spring

Spring

C O N

GRAY WHALE MIGRATION CORRIDOR

SB2

N

MN

16°

1953

0 MILES 1

See Map SB2b

Concepcion

Lighthouse

Spring

Point Conception

Government Point

Tour SB2: Jalama Beach Park to Gaviota Beach State Park

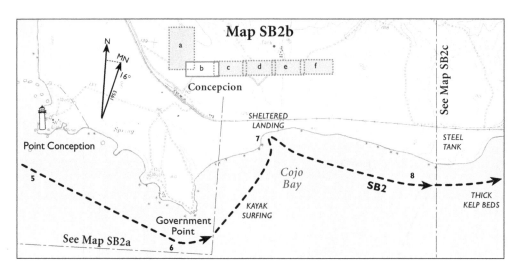

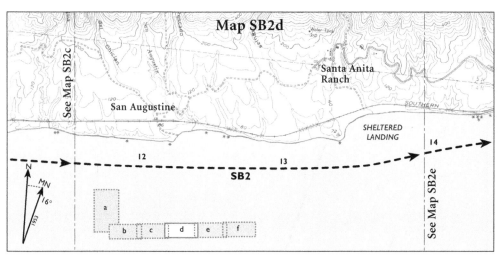

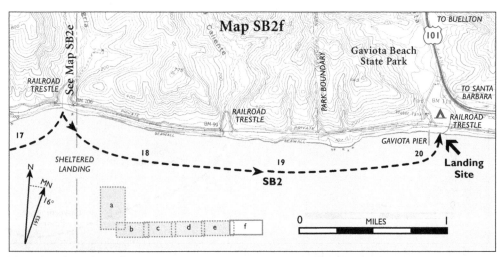

Tour SB2 (continued)

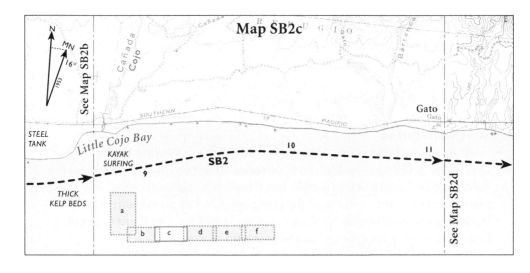

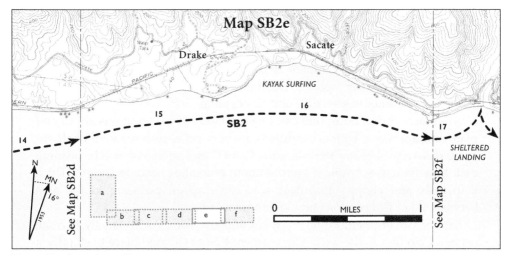

Tour SB2 (continued)

westerly in the afternoon. Strong, northerly Santa Ana winds sometimes blow during the afternoon and evening, making it difficult to paddle. Stay close to shore during a Santa Ana to avoid being blown to sea. Always check the weather forecast before launching and never attempt this trip if strong winds or waves are predicted.

Public access

Most of the property between Jalama Beach and Gaviota State Park is privately owned.

Kayak surfing

The coastline between Point Conception and Gaviota is noted for its good surfing waves.

Launching

Launch from the beach adjacent to Jalama Beach Park. Launching is possible only during periods when the waves are very small; usually during summer and early fall. A surf launch is almost always necessary.

Tour description

From Jalama Beach Park proceed toward Point Conception which is about five miles southeast. Paddle well offshore to avoid shoals and breaking waves. Point Conception is a bold headland on a relatively wide, low-lying marine terrace. From a distance the point appears like an offshore island. On the top of the headland is an old Coast Guard station. The Point Conception lighthouse stands on a rocky bluff near the tip of the point.

The Chumash Indians referred to Point Conception as the "Western Gate" and considered all land visible from the point to be sacred. According to legend, anyone who disturbed the land would face disaster. The point is a major bend in the California coastline where warm ocean currents coming from the south meet with the cold southward flowing California Current. This complex mixture creates an environment that includes plants and animals of both southern and northern species. During winter and spring, California gray whales are commonly seen off Point Conception.

Approach Point Conception cautiously. Observe the conditions ahead and plan your approach. Unless conditions are very calm, pass seaward of all offshore rocks and shoals. After rounding Point Conception, you will be heading east. Low-lying Government Point is about one mile ahead on the left. Thick kelp beds and choppy turbulent seas can impede paddling in the area between Point Conception and Government Point.

East of Government Point the wind and the waves will usually become calmer. Cojo Bay, in the lee of Government Point is a good place to stop for a lunch break. Cojo, named after a Chumash chieftain, has served as a haven for weary mariners for thousands of years. Land in the northeast corner of the bay in the shelter of the low bluff, which offers protection from the wind. The waves are usually small, but a surf landing may be necessary. The waves off Government Point are noted for good surfing.

From Cojo Bay head east around the point with a large steel tank on top. Little Cojo Bay, east of the point, is noted for good surfing. Thick offshore kelp beds can make paddling difficult. For smoother seas, paddle in the open water between the kelp beds and the mainland.

The coastline between Cojo and Gaviota consists of long, narrow, sand beaches backed by steep, low-lying bluffs. The marine terrace is about one-quarter mile wide. Runoff from the Santa Ynez Mountains, to the north, has eroded deep canyons across the level marine terrace. Sheltered landings can be found in the lee of most headlands. Occasional homes are visible on the hilltops and bluffs overlooking the water. These homes are all within the Hollister Ranch, a private community that stretches all the way to Gaviota State Park. Trespassing is prohibited on Hollister Ranch property.

The water is usually calm, clear and warm compared to the water north of Point Conception. Diving and fishing are excellent. Harbor seals, California sea lions, dolphins, and a wide variety of sea birds are commonly seen. Gray whales stop to rest in the calm, warm waters during their northern migration.

Gaviota State Beach can be easily identified by the pier and tall railroad trestle that spans Gaviota Canyon.

Landing
Land on the sand beach just east of the Gaviota Pier. The waves are usually small and break near the shore, but a surf landing may be necessary. The parking lot is adjacent to the beach.

What to do afterward
Day-use facilities and hiking trails are available at Gaviota Beach State Park. The historic Mission Santa Ynez is located east of Solvang on Highway 246.

Alternate tour: SB3

For more information
Jalama Beach Park (805) 736-3504
Regional Park Headquarters, Gaviota Beach State Park (805) 968-3294

TOUR SB3 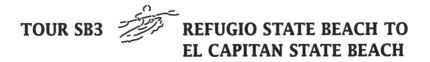 REFUGIO STATE BEACH TO EL CAPITAN STATE BEACH

Tour Details	
Skill level:	Beginner
Trip length/type:	6.0 miles; round-trip; open-ocean; two to three hours
Chart/map:	NOAA Chart #18721; USGS *Tajiguas* 7.5 min series

Summary
Calm seas and warm sand beaches await you on this relatively short and easy paddle, perfect for the beginner.

How to get there

To reach the launch site exit, Highway 101 at Refugio State Beach. Parking, restrooms, picnic facilities, and seasonal lifeguard services are available. Fee.

Camping

Camping is available at Refugio State Beach. For camping reservations, call ParkNet (800) 444-7275.

Hazards

Northerly Santa Ana winds sometimes blow during the afternoon and evening, making it difficult to paddle. Stay close to shore during a Santa Ana to avoid being blown to sea. Large waves can be encountered during the winter months. Always be prepared for the possibility of fog.

Public access

The shoreline between Refugio State Beach and El Capitan State Beach is accessible to the public.

Kayak surfing

Refugio Beach and El Capitan Beach are both well known for good surfing waves.

Launching

The parking lot is adjacent to the sand beach. Conditions are usually calm, but a surf launch may be necessary.

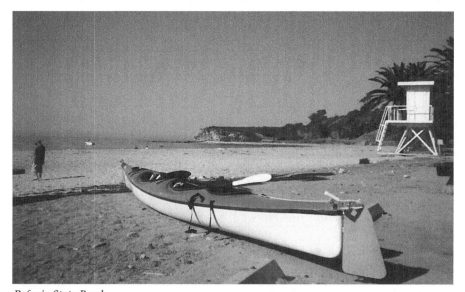

Refugio State Beach

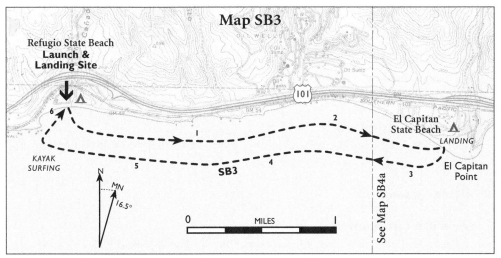

Tour SB3: Refugio State Beach to El Capitan State Beach

Tour description

Head east from Refugio cove. The rocky headlands are separated by narrow sand beaches. The bluff top is vegetated with coastal sage and scrub brush. To the north lie the Santa Ynez Mountains. The marine terrace is level and about one-quarter mile wide. A bluff-top bike path connects Refugio and El Capitan State Beaches. Several pathways lead from the bike path to the beach. The Southern Pacific Railroad and Highway 101 parallel the coastline just inland of the bike path. El Capitan Point is the forested headland that lies about three miles ahead.

The water is usually very clear and the sea floor is visible at depths of 15-20 feet. Harbor seals, California sea lions and dolphins, are occasionally seen. During winter and spring California gray whales pass close to shore.

The beach broadens and the bluff increases in height as you approach El Capitan Point. A lifeguard tower stands on the top of the headland and there are several lifeguard stations along the beach during the summer. Land on the sand beach just west of the point. A surf landing may be necessary. The beach on the east side of the point is covered with large, rounded boulders and cobbles and has good waves for surfing.

Picnic facilities, restrooms, and a food store are available on the bluff top just a short walk from the beach. El Capitan Creek, which discharges near the end of the point, supports a lush, forested riparian community. Monarch butterflies cluster on the trees during their breeding season in the fall. Archeological excavations revealed the remains of an ancient Chumash Indian village near the mouth of the creek.

From El Capitan Point return to Refugio State Beach. You may encounter a headwind during the afternoon.

Landing
Land on the beach where you launched. Conditions are usually calm but a surf landing may be necessary.

What to do afterward
Picnic facilities, biking trails, and hiking trails are available at Refugio State Beach.

Alternate tour: SB5

For more information
Regional Park Headquarters, Gaviota State Park (805) 968-3294

TOUR SB4   EL CAPITAN STATE BEACH TO GOLETA BEACH COUNTY PARK

Tour Details	
Skill level:	Advanced
Trip length/type:	13.8 miles; one-way; open-ocean; five to six hours
Chart/map:	NOAA Chart #18721; USGS *Tajiguas, Dos Pueblos,* and *Goleta* 7.5 min series

Summary
Secluded white sand beaches and good waves for kayak surfing can be found on this very remote section of coastline, most of which is accessible only by boat.

How to get there
To reach the launch site, exit Highway 101 at El Capitan State Beach. Parking, restrooms, picnic facilities, and seasonal lifeguard services are available. Fee.

To reach the landing site, exit Highway 101 at Fairview Avenue. Drive south about one mile to Fowler Road and go right to Wm. L. Moffett Place. Go left at Moffett Place, which becomes Sand Spit Road. Turn right at Goleta Beach County Park. Parking, restrooms, picnic facilities, and seasonal lifeguard services are available. No fee.

Camping

Camping is available at El Capitan State Beach. For camping reservations, call ParkNet (800) 444-7275.

Hazards

This tour is located in a remote area with limited access to the beach; be well prepared. Strong northerly Santa Ana winds sometimes blow during the afternoon and evening, making it difficult to paddle. Stay close to shore during a Santa Ana to avoid being blown to sea. Strong swells can be encountered during the winter months. Always be prepared for the possibility of fog. A very shallow reef extends for nearly a mile off Naples Point. Choppy conditions, strong currents, and breaking waves are common on the reef. A shallow reef also extends off Coal Oil Point. In the vicinity of Naples Point, the water is often covered with an oil slick which can be very messy and smelly.

Public access

Most of the shoreline between El Capitan Beach and Coal Oil Point is privately owned and inaccessible to the public; from Coal Oil Point to Goleta Beach is accessible.

Kayak surfing

El Capitan Beach, Naples Reef, Coal Oil Point, and Goleta Point (Campus Point) are all well known for good surfing waves.

Launching

Launch from the beach on the west side of the El Capitan Point. Conditions are usually calm but a surf launch may be necessary.

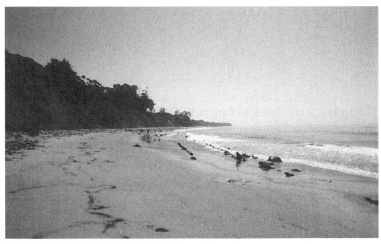

Secluded beach west of Naples Point

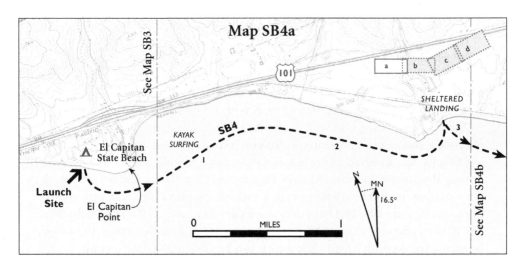

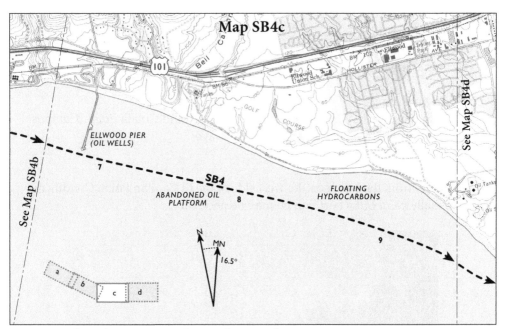

Tour SB4: El Capitan State Beach to Goleta Beach

Tour description

Head east from El Capitan Beach. Naples Point with its abrupt bluff and very distinctive flat top is located about five miles southeast. Between El Capitan Point and Naples Point is a long, relatively straight stretch of coastline with a high vertical bluff and a narrow sandy beach. The coastline faces southwest and is sheltered, with numerous good landing spots. Highway 101 leads inland just east of El Capitan Point, and public access to the beach is limited until you reach Coal Oil Point.

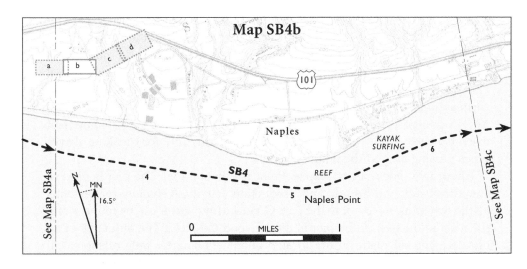

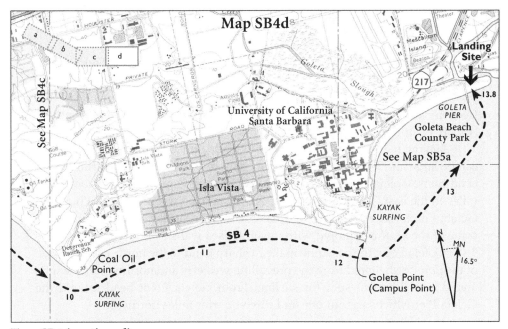

Tour SB4 (continued)

About half-way to Naples Point is a small, low-lying, rocky headland. This small point of land has a much less distinctive profile than Naples Point and is difficult to see from a distance. The west side of the point is piled high with driftwood and the east side is scattered with large, rounded boulders and cobbles. A sheltered landing can be found in the lee of the point.

East of the small point is another long, straight stretch of deserted beach with a high vertical bluff. The Southern Pacific railroad tracks run along the top of the bluff. Just west of Naples Point is Dos Pueblos Canyon, a narrow, steep-sided canyon spanned by the railroad trestle. On the beach at the mouth of the canyon is the wreck of a sailboat with a large hole in the side.

A short distance past Dos Pueblos Canyon is Naples Point. From Naples Point, on a clear day, it is possible to see all the way from Refugio Point to Coal Oil Point—a distance of about 15 miles. The bluff at Naples Point is high and steep and the marine terrace is very broad and flat. To the north lie the Santa Ynez Mountains and to the south, the Channel Islands. A very shallow reef extends nearly a mile off Naples Point. Watch carefully for breaking waves when passing around the point.

About two miles east of Naples Point is Ellwood Pier. The pier is used to support offshore oil drilling and production activity. A shallow reef extends all the way from the point to the pier. Good surfing waves can be found along the reef. To the east of the pier is the Ellwood Oil Field. The remnants of an old decaying oil platform are located about one-quarter mile offshore. Oil barges and oil-field service boats lie at anchor. There is a large amount of hydrocarbon floating on the water and the smell of oil is very strong. Be prepared for clean-up duties after the trip. Vegetable oil and a rag work well for removing the black goo.

Approximately one and one-half miles east of the Ellwood Oil Field is Coal Oil Point, a low-lying point of land. Sand dunes are visible northwest of the point. On the point is a building surrounded by trees. Protruding above the trees are the taller buildings of the University of California Santa Barbara (UCSB) campus. Stork Tower, in the center of the campus, is most prominent.

A shallow reef with thick kelp beds extends off Coal Oil Point. The waves can be large and break a long distance offshore. Avoid this reef during rough conditions. Goleta Point (also known as Campus Point) is visible about two miles to the east. The community of Isla Vista is between Coal Oil Point and Goleta Point. Extensive sea-cliff erosion is evident in the Isla Vista area, and some of the bluff is armored with unsightly sea walls.

At Goleta Point the coastline makes a sharp bend to the north. The east side of the point is sheltered from the prevailing westerly and northwesterly winds and is a well-known spot for surfing. From Goleta Point head toward the Goleta Pier which is about one and three-quarter miles northeast.

Landing

Land on the sand beach east of the pier at Goleta Beach County Park. Be careful to avoid the swimming areas, which are designated by a row of white buoys. Conditions are usually calm but a surf landing may be necessary.

What to do afterward

A snack bar and a restaurant are adjacent to the pier. The University of California Santa Barbara campus is about one mile west of the pier.

Alternate tour: SB5

For more information

Santa Barbara County, Department of Parks and Recreation (805) 568-2460
Goleta Chamber of Commerce (805) 967-4618

TOUR SB5 GOLETA BEACH COUNTY PARK TO ARROYO BURRO (HENDRY'S) BEACH COUNTY PARK

Tour Details	
Skill level:	Intermediate
Trip length/type:	5.4 miles; one-way; open ocean; two to three hours
Chart/map:	NOAA Chart #18721; USGS *Goleta* and *Santa Barbara* 7.5 min series

Summary

A scrumptious brunch awaits you at the Brown Pelican Restaurant at Arroyo Burro County Beach following your leisurely Sunday morning coastal excursion.

How to get there

To reach the launch site, exit Highway 101 at Fairview Avenue. Drive south about one mile to Fowler Road and go right to Wm. L. Moffett Place. Go left at Moffett Place, which becomes Sand Spit Road. Turn right at Goleta Beach County Park. Parking, restrooms, picnic facilities, telephone, a restaurant, and seasonal lifeguard services are available. No fee.

To reach the landing site, exit Highway 101 at Las Positas Road and proceed south about two miles to Cliff Drive. Turn right on Cliff Drive and go about two blocks to Arroyo Burro Beach County Park at 2981 Cliff Drive. Parking, restrooms, picnic facilities, telephone, and a restaurant, are available. No fee.

Camping

Camping is available at El Capitan State Beach, off Highway 101 about 12 miles north of Goleta Beach. For camping reservations, call ParkNet (800) 444-7275.

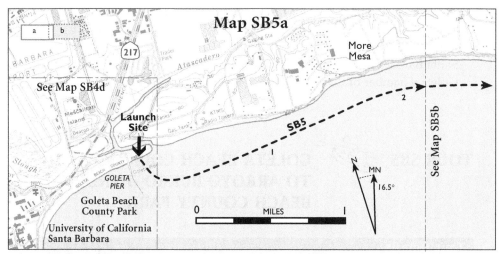

Tour SB5: Goleta Beach to Arroyo Burro (Hendry's) Beach

Hazards

Strong northerly Santa Ana winds can blow during the afternoon and evening, making it difficult to paddle. Stay close to shore during a Santa Ana to avoid being blown to sea. Large waves can be encountered during the winter months. Always be prepared for the possibility of fog. Localized thick kelp beds can make paddling difficult.

Public access

Most of the bluff top is privately owned. Beach access is limited to a few narrow paths leading down the steep bluff.

Kayak surfing

Goleta Point (Campus Point) is well known for good surfing waves.

Launching

Launch from the sand beach east of the pier at Goleta Beach County Park. Be careful to avoid the swimming areas, which are designated by a row of white buoys. Conditions are usually calm but a surf landing may be necessary

Tour description

From Goleta Beach, head east. The marine terrace is wide and relatively level. The Santa Ynez Mountains are visible to the north, and the Channel Islands, several miles offshore to the south, can be seen on a clear day. East of Goleta Beach are the white bluffs of More Mesa, an area occupied for thousands of years by the Chumash Indians. Today elegant homes surrounded by tall eucalyptus trees are located along the bluff top. A narrow, white-sand beach stretches along the shoreline.

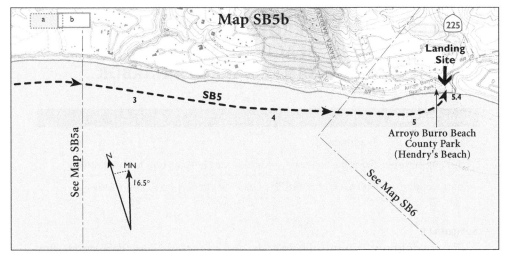

Tour SB5 (continued)

Several shallow reefs with thick kelp beds extend up to three-quarter mile offshore. The sandy beach is relatively straight and narrow, backed by a high vertical bluff. Access to the beach from the bluff top is limited to a few narrow stairways and footpaths.

Water visibility is usually good and the rocky reefs are well known for fishing and scuba diving. In 1977, 25,000 tires were dumped into the ocean about 800 yards off Arroyo Burro, creating an artificial reef in about 60 feet of water. Dolphins, California sea lions, and harbor seals are frequently seen in this area, and California gray whales can be spotted from December through March. Fishing is good for kelp bass, and rock fish. Arroyo Burro is a narrow canyon about two miles east of Santa Barbara Point. A flat-roofed restaurant with large, square windows is visible on the beach west of the creek.

Landing

Land on the beach adjacent to the parking area at Arroyo Burro County Beach. Avoid designated swimming areas, identified by white buoys. Conditions are usually calm, but a surf landing may be necessary.

What to do afterward

Arroyo Burro is a beautiful setting with a sandy beach, volleyball courts, a natural stream habitat, picnic facilities, and a restaurant.

Alternate tour: SB7

For more information

Goleta Chamber of Commerce (805) 967-4618
Santa Barbara County, Department of Parks and Recreation (805) 568-2460

TOUR SB6 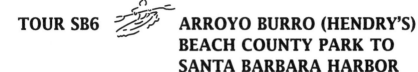 ARROYO BURRO (HENDRY'S) BEACH COUNTY PARK TO SANTA BARBARA HARBOR

Tour Details

Skill level:	Beginner
Trip length/type:	5.0 miles; one-way; open-ocean/harbor; two to three hours
Chart/map:	NOAA Chart #18721; USGS *Santa Barbara* 7.5 min series

Summary

Playful dolphins, bountiful kelp beds, and a bustling Santa Barbara Harbor are just a few of the sights you can expect on this relatively short tour.

How to get there

To reach the launch site, exit Highway 101 at Las Positas Road and proceed south about two miles to Cliff Drive. Turn right on Cliff Drive and go about two blocks to Arroyo Burro Beach County Park at 2981 Cliff Drive. Parking, restrooms, picnic facilities, telephone, and a restaurant, are available. No fee.

To reach the landing site, exit Highway 101 at Castillo Street. Go about one-half mile south (toward the harbor) to Cabrillo Boulevard. Turn right on Cabrillo Boulevard and go to Harbor Way. Turn left on Harbor Way and then immediately turn left again into the Santa Barbara Harbor parking lot. The launch ramp is at the east end of the lot. Restrooms are available. Fee.

Camping

Camping is available at El Capitan State Beach located off Highway 101 approximately 15 miles north of Arroyo Burro Beach. For camping reservations, call ParkNet (800) 444-7275.

Hazards

Strong, northerly Santa Ana winds sometimes blow during the afternoon and evening, making it difficult to paddle. Stay close to shore during a Santa Ana to avoid being blown to sea. Large waves may be encountered during the winter months. Always be prepared for the possibility of fog. Localized thick kelp beds can make paddling difficult in the vicinity of Santa Barbara Point. Choppy seas may be encountered outside Santa Barbara Harbor due to boat traffic and waves being reflected off the breakwater. Boat traffic can be congested; always follow the rules of the road.

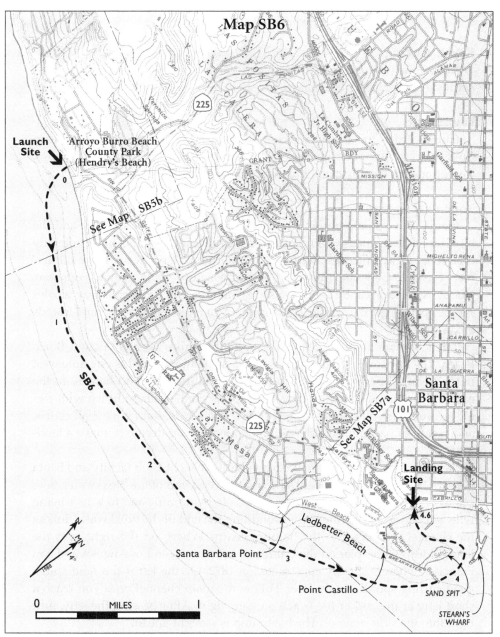

Tour SB6: Arroyo Burro Beach County Park (Hendry's Beach) to Santa Barbara Harbor

Public access

Most of the bluff top is privately owned. Beach access is limited to a few narrow paths leading down the steep bluff. Plenty of parking and easy beach access are available at Ledbetter Beach, just west of the harbor.

Kayak surfing

During the winter, good surfing waves can be found at the sand spit off the entrance to Santa Barbara Harbor.

Launching

Launch from the beach adjacent to the parking area at Arroyo Burro County Beach. Avoid designated swimming areas, identified by white buoys. Conditions are usually calm, but a surf landing may be necessary.

Tour description

From Arroyo Burro Beach head east. The bluff is high and steep, and the bluff top is developed with homes. The narrow sand beach is interrupted by occasional rocky outcrops. During calm conditions, landing spots are numerous. The kelp beds are thick and extend a considerable distance offshore. Dolphins, sea lions and harbor seals are common, and California gray whales can be spotted during winter and spring. On a clear day the Channel Islands are visible.

Santa Barbara Point is located about three miles east of Arroyo Burro Beach. The low tower of the Santa Barbara navigational light is one mile west of the point. The tower is difficult to spot amid the trees and homes. To the east of the point is Ledbetter Beach, a popular Santa Barbara beach with picnic facilities, fire pits, showers, restrooms, snack bars, sand volleyball courts, and plenty of parking. Avoid swimming areas if you decide to make a landing.

East of Ledbetter Beach are the Santa Barbara Yacht Club facility and Santa Barbara Harbor. The harbor entrance is at the east end of the breakwater. Seas can be choppy off the harbor entrance due to boat traffic and to waves being reflected off the breakwater. After rounding the end of the breakwater, follow the channel markers into the harbor. Stearns Wharf, on the right, was the longest deep-water pier on the California coast between Los Angeles and San Francisco when originally constructed in 1872. On the left is the sand spit, a good surfing spot during winter. Follow the main channel until you reach a short jetty at the end of the beach on your right. After passing the jetty, turn right into the side channel. The boat ramp is straight ahead.

Landing

Land at the public boat ramp at the marina in Santa Barbara Harbor. There is a finger pier for loading and unloading gear.

What to do afterward

Harbor facilities include gift shops, restaurants, and marine supplies. The harbor master's office is located above the Chandlery. A walkway and bike path extend along the water front. Of historical interest are the Santa Barbara Mission, founded in 1786, and the Museum of Natural History. Marine resources of the Channel Islands are on exhibit at the Sea Center on Stearns Wharf.

Alternate tour: LA3

For more information

Santa Barbara County, Department of Parks and Recreation (805) 568-2460
Santa Barbara Harbor Patrol (805) 564-5530
Santa Barbara Waterfront Business (805) 564-5520

TOUR SB7 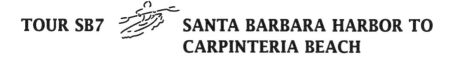 SANTA BARBARA HARBOR TO CARPINTERIA BEACH

Tour Details	
Skill level:	Intermediate
Trip length/type:	11.0 miles; one-way; open ocean; three to four hours
Chart/map:	NOAA Chart #18725; USGS *Santa Barbara* and *Carpinteria* 7.5 min series

Summary

Do you ever wonder what the rich and famous residents of Montecito see out of their living-room window? They'll be sure to see *you* as you paddle along this section of coast developed with multi-million dollar ocean-front mansions.

How to get there

To reach the launch site, exit Highway 101 at Castillo Street. Go about one-half mile south (toward the harbor) to Cabrillo Boulevard. Turn right on Cabrillo Boulevard and go to Harbor Way. Turn left on Harbor Way and then immediately turn left again into the Santa Barbara Harbor parking lot. The launch ramp is at the east end of the lot. Restrooms are available. Fee.

To reach the landing site coming from the north, exit Highway 101 at Linden Avenue. Proceed west (toward the beach) about three-quarter mile to Sandyland Street. Go right on Sandyland to Ash Avenue, turn left and park at the end of the street. To reach the landing site coming from the south, exit Highway 101 at Casitas Pass Road and go one block west to Carpinteria Avenue. Go right on Carpinteria Avenue to Linden Avenue and go left on Linden Avenue to Sandyland Street. Go right on Sandyland to Ash Avenue, turn left and park at the end of the street. Street parking, restrooms, and seasonal lifeguard services are available. There is no fee.

Camping

Camping is available at Carpinteria State Beach, at the end of Palm Avenue in Carpinteria. For camping reservations, call ParkNet (800) 444-7275.

Hazards

Boat traffic can be congested; always follow the rules of the road. Stay clear of designated swimming areas off East Beach, Fernald Cove, Summerland Beach, and Carpinteria Beach. The coastline between Loon Point and Sand Point is exposed to westerly winds and waves, so be prepared for the possibility of increased wind and chop. Sand Point is a low-lying headland with a shallow reef extending nearly one mile offshore; submerged rocks, thick kelp beds, and breaking waves can be hazardous. Strong northerly Santa Ana winds sometimes blow during the afternoon and evening, making it difficult to paddle. Stay close to shore during a Santa Ana to avoid being blown to sea. Always be prepared for the possibility of fog.

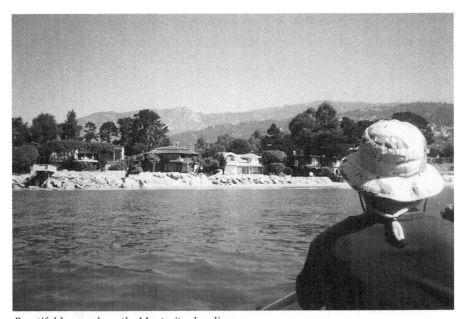

Beautiful homes along the Montecito shoreline

Public access
Public access is available at East Beach, Butterfly Beach, Summerland Beach, and Carpinteria Beach.

Kayak surfing
During the winter, good surfing waves can be found at the sand spit off the entrance to Santa Barbara Harbor, and Fernald (Hammonds) Point.

Launching
Launch from the boat ramp at the marina in Santa Barbara Harbor. There is a finger pier for loading and unloading gear.

Tour description
From the launch site follow the main channel to Stearns Wharf, then head east. Be sure to stay outside the designated swimming areas along East Beach. On the left are several large waterfront hotels and the Cabrillo Pavilion Bathhouse, built in 1925.

About one and one-half miles east of Stearns Wharf, the beach merges into a low bluff which extends for about one mile. On the bluff overlooking the beach is the Santa Barbara Cemetery. The trees on the cemetery grounds have been sculptured into an interesting variety of shapes and sizes which stand out clearly against the sky.

East of the cemetery is Edgecliff Point, a low-lying headland. The Biltmore Hotel and the prominent white tower of the Coral Casino on Edgecliff Point can be seen from well offshore. To the east of Edgecliff Point is a small, protected cove. Several homes are clustered on the beach at the west end of the cove, and the Miramar Hotel with its distinctive blue roof is located at the cove's east end. The water in the cove is shallow and the seafloor is clearly visible through the thick, green sea grass. East of the Miramar Hotel is Fernald Point (also known as Hammonds Point), well known for its good surfing waves.

Directly ahead and rising abruptly is Ortega Hill. Highway 101 with its ceaseless flow of cars is visible leading up the west side of the hill. Downslope from the highway is the Southern Pacific railroad. A large sea wall has been constructed along the base of the hill in an attempt to slow the inevitable retreat of the shoreline.

East of Ortega Hill is the small beach community of Summerland. Lookout County Park, with restrooms and a picnic area is located at the top of the bluff. A public path leads from the park to the beach. The bluff is relatively high and the beach is long and narrow. The waves are usually small, and landing a kayak is possible during most of the year. Avoid the designated swimming areas.

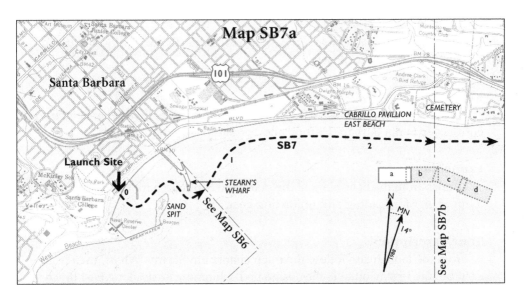

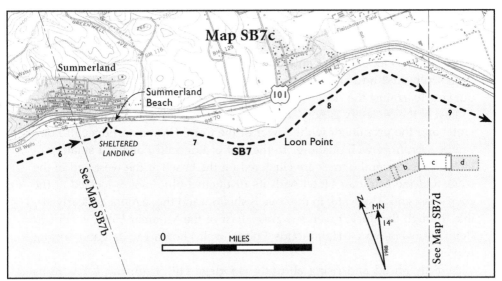

Tour SB7: Santa Barbara Harbor to Carpinteria Beach

In 1896, the world's first offshore oil well was drilled off the end of a pier at Summerland. By 1906, more than 400 wells had been drilled off the beaches of Summerland. Platform Hazel, the first offshore oil-drilling platform, was erected two miles offshore in 1958. Today numerous offshore platforms are visible from the shore.

At the east end of Summerland Beach and approximately seven and one-half miles east of Santa Barbara Harbor is Loon Point. A forest of eucalyptus

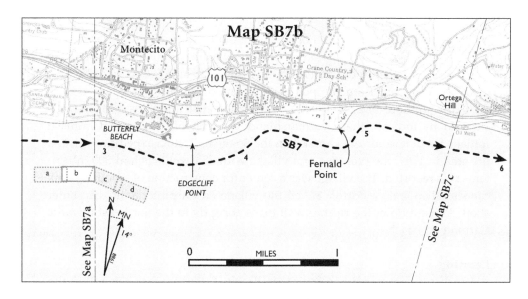

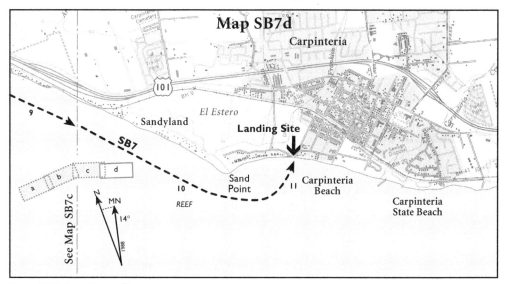

Tour SB7 (continued)

and cypress trees on the point provides habitat for the migratory Monarch butterfly. The bluff is reddish-brown and is slightly higher in elevation on the west side of the point. The sandy beach is narrow with numerous rocky outcrops; a thick kelp forest extends far offshore. On the east side of the point overlooking the calm waters are several beautiful residences.

A low-lying sand spit extends from Loon Point about two and one-half miles southeast to Sand Point. A massive rip-rap sea wall has been constructed to protect the homes along the beach. Santa's Village, a commercial development on the west side of Sand Point, is a well-known Highway 101 landmark.

Sand Point is a low headland with a shallow reef extending nearly one mile offshore. Submerged rocks, thick kelp beds, and breaking waves can be hazardous. Just inland from the point is Carpinteria Marsh, a 230-acre coastal lagoon. Thousands of migratory birds visit the marsh annually. Archeological excavations indicate that the marshland was inhabited by the Chumash Indians for thousands of years. When the Spanish, Portola expedition, visited the area in 1769, the presence of a village with 38 dwellings and 300 inhabitants was reported. The village was a center for construction of wooden plank canoes called *tomols*. Portola called the village La Carpinteria, the carpenter shop. At Sand Point the rip-rap wall turns abruptly to the northeast towards Carpinteria Beach.

Landing

Land at the west end of Carpinteria Beach. The waves are generally calm but a surf landing may be necessary. Avoid designated swimming areas, identified by white buoys.

What to do afterward

Downtown Carpinteria is about four blocks east of the landing site.

Alternate tour: LA3

For more information

Santa Barbara Harbor Patrol (805) 564-5530
Santa Barbara Harbor Waterfront Business (805) 564-5520
City of Carpinteria (805) 684-5405

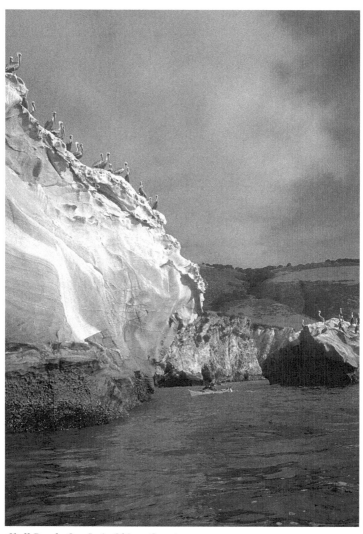

Shell Beach, San Luis Obispo County

Channel Island Tours

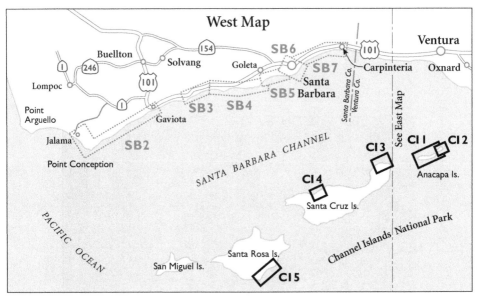

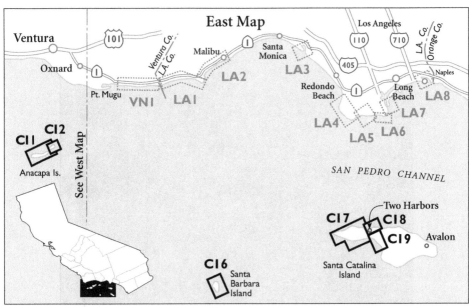

Tour		Skill Level	Length
CI1:	Anacapa: Landing Cove to West End	Advanced	11.2 miles
CI2:	Anacapa: Landing Cove to Pinniped Point	Beginner	2.7 miles
CI3:	Santa Cruz: Scorpion Bay to Cavern Point	Beginner	3.5 miles
CI4:	Santa Cruz: Cueva Valdez to Arch Rock	Intermediate	4.7 miles
CI5:	Santa Rosa: Ford Point to Johnson's Lee	Intermediate	4.0 miles
CI6:	Santa Barbara: Circumnavigation	Intermediate	6.0 miles
CI7:	Santa Catalina: Isthmus Cove to Catalina Harbor	Advanced	17.5 miles
CI8:	Santa Catalina: Isthmus Cove to Blue Cavern Point	Beginner	4.8 miles
CI9:	Santa Catalina: Catalina Harbor to Little Harbor	Advanced	9.7 miles

Chapter 5

The Channel Islands

Our group had just spent three wonderful days touring Santa Barbara island. I said goodbye to the park ranger as I passed by the visitor center for the last time. He was a great host and had been very helpful during our brief stay. It took three trips to haul my camping gear from the campsite to the pier at Landing Cove. As I walked down the steep path to the pier, I reflected on our many adventures.

The first day, after a three-hour channel crossing on the Island Packer's Jeffrey Arvid *we set up camp and then went for a paddle around the island. The island is only a mile wide so a complete circumnavigation only took about four hours. The adventure exceeded all my expectations; sea lions and elephant seals, sea caves, crystal clear water, kelp forests, more sea lions, blow holes, and more sea lions. At night the sky was clear and there were a million stars. It was so clear we could even see the lights of the mainland over 40 miles away. All night long we could hear the distant barking of sea lions.*

The next morning the wind was howling. It was unsafe to paddle so the park ranger took us on tour of the island. From Signal Peak, the highest point on the island, we were able to see almost all the other Channel Islands and the mainland. The wind continued to blow through the evening but we had a good time telling stories and watching the constellations move across the night sky.

We awakened to a spectacular sunrise over Santa Catalina Island, which lies 20 miles to the west. The wind was calm and we were all anxious to be on the water again. After breakfast we launched our kayaks and paddled to Sutil Island, a large rock about one-half mile southwest of Santa Barbara Island. The sky was clear and the water was smooth as glass. Along the way we were escorted by frisky sea lion pups that seemed very interested in our colorful kayaks.

But now it was finally time to leave. I was sad as I walked down the steep trail to the landing. By the time I reached the dock I was hot and tired. I knew we only had a short time before we were scheduled to depart but the water looked inviting and I felt like one last swim. I dove into the cool refreshing water. As I swam away from the dock, I soon realized that I wasn't alone. I was surrounded by about 20 frisky sea lion pups eager for a good time. They swam circles around me, jumped into the air and occasionally would brush gently against my side. One in particular kept popping up in front of me with a twinkle in his eye and seemed to be smiling. We played together for about 20 minutes until I heard the loud diesel engines of the Jeffrey Arvid *roar to life. I bade farewell to my new friends and reluctantly swam slowly back to the dock.*

— Santa Barbara Island, October 20, 1996

TOUR CI1 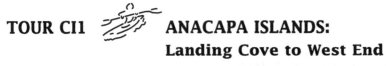 ANACAPA ISLANDS:
Landing Cove to West End

Tour Details

Skill level:	Advanced
Trip length/type:	11.2 miles; round-trip; open-ocean; five to seven hours (depending on how many caves you want to explore)
Chart/map:	NOAA Chart #18729; USGS *Anacapa Island* 7.5 min series

Summary
Your itinerary on this island adventure includes hundreds of spectacular sea caves, majestic geologic land forms, crystal-clear water, forests of giant kelp, sea lions, harbor seals, and a brown pelican rookery.

How to get there
The Anacapa Islands are three small islets located about 11.5 miles southwest of Oxnard and 16 miles south of Ventura. Daily excursions to Landing Cove at East Anacapa Island are available year-round through Island Packers and Truth Aquatics, the authorized concessionaires to the Channel Islands National Park. For information and reservations, call Island Packers at (805) 642-1393, or Truth Aquatics at (805) 963-3564.

Camping
A limited number of primitive campsites are available on East Anacapa Island. From the landing dock, a steep stairway (154 steps) leads to the top of the bluff, and then it is a one-half mile walk to the campsites. Backpacking equipment is recommended for transporting food and camping gear. Pit toilets and picnic tables are provided; bring your own water, windbreak, and shelter. Stake your tent well; it gets very windy. Open fires are prohibited. For reservations and permits contact the National Park Reservation System (800) 365-CAMP.

Hazards
Choppy seas are likely during the late afternoon from Cathedral Cave to Middle Anacapa and at the west end of West Anacapa. Shelter from the wind and chop can be found in the larger coves. Swift currents often flow between the islands and at the east and west ends of the chain. Dense fog is most common in June and July. Santa Ana winds can occur any time of the year but are most common from September to November. Wear a helmet and PFD, and

carry a waterproof flashlight when exploring the caves. In an emergency, park rangers can be reached by radio on Channel 16.

Public access

Landing is permitted on East Anacapa and Middle Anacapa island beaches. Access above the beaches at Middle Anacapa is with ranger escort only. Access above the beaches at East Anacapa Island is by way of the landing cove only. West Anacapa is a Research Natural Area, and no landings are permitted (except at Frenchy's Cove) without written permission from the park superintendent. From January 1 to October 31 the shoreline between Frenchy's cove and Portuguese Rock and out to a water depth of 120 feet (about 150 yards) are designated as the California Brown Pelican Fledgling Area and are closed to the public (check with the park ranger for the current regulations). The waters on the north shore of East Anacapa down to a depth of 60 feet are designated as a "natural area." To remove any type of aquatic life from this area is prohibited. Landing is prohibited on offshore rocks and islets. This tour is located within the Channel Islands National Marine Sanctuary.

Kayak surfing

The Anacapa Islands are not noted for good surfing waves.

Launching

From the dock at Landing Cove on Anacapa, kayaks must be lowered 10-12 feet to the water with a hoist. Maximum capacity of the hoist is 300 pounds, and extra line should be brought along to rig a lifting bridle to attach your

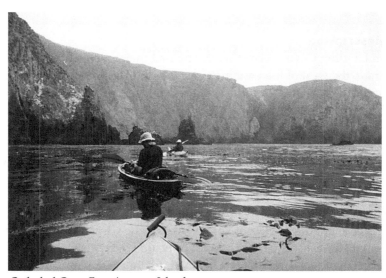

Cathedral Cove, East Anacapa Island

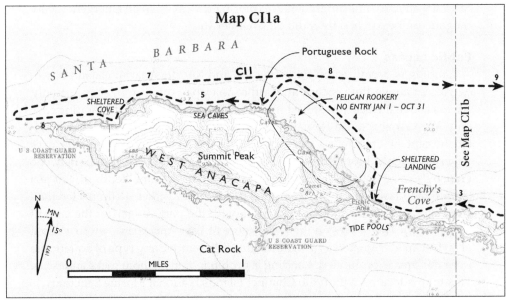

Tour CI1: Anacapa Islands—Landing Cove to West End

kayak to the hoist. It's best to load your kayak before lowering it to the water so you don't have to load a boat which is moving up and down with the surge. Launching a kayak with a hoist is a two- to three-person job. A steel ladder extends from the dock to the water. Negotiating the last step from the bottom of the ladder into your kayak can be difficult when there is a strong surge.

Tour description

From Landing Cove proceed west. The first major attraction as you round the point to the west of the Landing Cove is a blow hole that can send a spout of water into the air like a California gray whale if the tide and swell are just right. The precipitous bluff is about 50 to 100 feet in height and drops steeply to the water offering few landing spots. Spewed from an ancient submarine volcano, the molten lava flowed along the seafloor until it cooled. The solidified rock was subsequently uplifted and exposed to the pounding waves which sculptured the large caverns, blow holes, and spectacular arches we see today.

The name Anacapa is derived from the Chumash word "Eneepah" which means ever changing or deceptive. Perhaps as the Chumash traveled to the islands in their *tomol* canoes, the islands appeared deceptively large. Anacapa is the only Channel Island that has retained its Chumash name. Although it is believed that the Chumash didn't have a permanent settlement on the

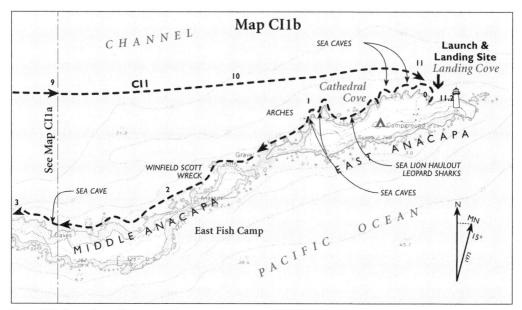

Map CI1b

Tour CI1 (continued)

Anacapa Islands, they did make frequent stops to hunt fish and gather shell-fish. Piles of broken shell and bone fragments called middens are the only visible remnants of their presence.

Between the cries of gulls and the barking of sea lions, the foghorn which can be heard from just about everywhere on the island provides an ominous warning for ships to stay clear of this magnificent, yet barren island. Many ships have met their doom on the treacherous rocks.

The first lighthouse on the island, built in 1912, was an unmanned beacon on a 50 foot metal tower. The original lighthouse was replaced in 1932. The new lighthouse was manned by a Coast Guard staff of 4 persons who lived with their families on the island. In 1967, the lighthouse was automated and most of the original buildings for the lighthouse keepers were removed. The remaining buildings are used to house park service personnel. The original lighthouse lamp with its beautiful glass work is on display at the visitor center.

About one-half mile west of the Landing Cove is Cathedral Cove. Private yachts frequently anchor in the shelter of the bay. Several sea lions live in a large cave on the east side of the cove. The curious pups are always eager to greet newcomers. The guano-covered rocks and bluffs overlooking the cove are crowded with cormorants and brown pelicans. The kelp forest is thick and the water a deep blue. Bright orange garabaldi and spotted leopard sharks can be seen swimming along the bottom. Don't be afraid; the leopard sharks are harmless.

A large cavern passes through the point on the west side of the cove. Beyond is another small headland penetrated by a labyrinth of caves known as Cathedral Caves. Inside the caves, you feel as if you were in a cathedral. Two large pillars support the middle chamber with smaller alcoves on either side. Surging waves echo off the cavern's walls. The air is damp and misty and the water a glowing emerald green. If you have a mask and fins, try snorkeling through the caves.

From Cathedral Cave to Middle Anacapa is about one-half mile. The two islands are separated by a channel with shallow reefs and exposed rocks. During a south swell, there can be strong currents and breaking waves in the channel.

Middle Anacapa has a similar appearance to East Anacapa, with steep vertical bluffs and a flat wave-cut terrace above. Shallow tide pools just deep enough to paddle your kayak across are covered with a carpet of bright purple sea urchins. Offshore lies the wreck of the side-wheel steamer, *Winfield Scott* which ran aground in the fog on the night of December 2, 1853. The 250 passengers waited for 8 days on the barren shore of Middle Anacapa until they were finally rescued.

Middle and West Anacapa are separated by a very narrow channel of water. Frenchy's Cove, located at the eastern tip of West Anacapa is the best landing on the island. Frenchy's was named after Raymond Ledreaux, a Frenchman who migrated to the Anacapa Islands after his wife died from a flu epidemic in 1918. Frenchy's hut was a favorite gathering spot for local fishermen and boaters. Because there was no adequate source of fresh water on the island, Frenchy collected rainwater and stored it in drums. Indian Water Cave, just west of Frenchy's Cove, is the island's only source of fresh water. A slow trickle of water which drips from the ceiling of the cave is collected in a natural basin in the rock. The cave is accessible only from the sea. Chumash Indians who stopped at the island are believed to have used this as their water source. In 1954 at age 68, Frenchy was moved to the mainland after living for 26 years on the island.

Although hiking is prohibited on Middle and West Anacapa without written permission from the park superintendent, you may land at Frenchy's Cove to explore the beautiful tide pools on the south side of the island. The tide pools are filled with a variety of marine organisms including sea stars, octopus, eels, mussels, barnacles, urchins, sea anemone, and hermit crabs. At a low tide it's possible to observe the different environments of the intertidal zones. The ability of each species to live in a particular zone depends on its tolerance to air as well as sunlight and food source. Highest on the rocks, in the splash zone which is only submerged at high tide, are limpets, chitons, and acorn barnacles. Farther out on the reef, in the middle intertidal zone which is usually submerged twice a day, are mussels, and gooseneck barnacles. The lowest intertidal zone is usually only exposed to the air at the lowest tides and supports the greatest variety of marine life forms including sea stars, sea anenome, sea urchins, snails, hermit crabs, and abalone. Because Anacapa is an ecological reserve, marine life is protected; nothing may be taken or possessed.

From Frenchy's Cove continue towards Portuguese Rock. From January 1 to October 31 the shoreline between Frenchy's cove and Portuguese Rock as well as the waters to about 150 yards offshore are designated as the California Brown Pelican Fledgling Area and are closed to the public (check with the park ranger for the current regulations). Be sure to paddle well offshore during the restricted months. Unlike low-lying and flat topped East and Middle Anacapa, West Anacapa has a sharp ridge that runs the entire length of the island. Summit Peak, elevation 936 feet, is the highest point on the Anacapa Islands.

In the lee of Portuguese Rock there are several interesting caves. One is nearly 300 feet in length with a ceiling height of up to 20 feet. The caverns are extensive with several chambers. From Portuguese Rock to the west end of West Anacapa are several more caves but the shoreline is exposed to the prevailing wind and waves and access is difficult. Approximately one-half mile from the west end is a sheltered cove offering good protection from a westerly wind. Dive boats often anchor in the cove.

The west end of the island is a sharp finger of land trending due west. Currents are strong and breaking waves are common on the shoals. Santa Cruz Island, five miles west of Anacapa, is visible on a clear day.

Return to Landing Cove along either the north or the south side of the islands, depending on the conditions. During the summer, strong south swells can make paddling on the south side of the island uncomfortable. The prevailing westerly wind will provide a following wind and sea for the return journey.

Landing

Land at the dock at Landing Cove. To Hoist your kayak from the water to the dock will require two people. From the water, one person attaches the bridle to the kayak while the other operates the hoist. Boats may not remain tied to the dock. Storage of kayaks on the dock should be coordinated with the park ranger.

What to do afterward

East Anacapa has a visitor center with displays and one and one-half miles of hiking trails. On a clear day, the hike offers breathtaking views of the entire island and its magnificent coastline. A trail guide is available at the visitor center. Due to the fragile environment, hiking is limited to the well-marked trails and collecting of cultural and natural resources is prohibited.

Alternate tour: CI2

For more information
Island Packers (805) 642-1393
Channel Islands National Park Visitors Center (805) 658-5730;
    www.nips.gov/chis
Channel Islands National Marine Sanctuary (805) 966-7107

TOUR CI2 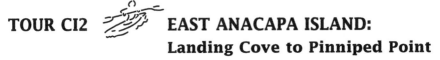 EAST ANACAPA ISLAND:
Landing Cove to Pinniped Point

Tour Details

Skill level:	Beginner
Trip length/type:	2.7 miles; round-trip;open-ocean; two to three hours
Chart/map:	NOAA Chart #18729; USGS *Anacapa Island* 7.5 min series

Summary
This tour offers breathtaking views of Arch Rock and a visit to the California sea lion haul-out at Pinniped Point located on the south side of East Anacapa Island.

How to get there
East Anacapa Island is about 11.5 miles southwest of Oxnard and 16 miles south of Ventura. Daily excursions to Landing Cove at East Anacapa Island are available year-round through Island Packers and Truth Aquatics, the authorized concessionaires to the Channel Islands National Park. For information and reservations, call Island Packers at (805) 642-1393, or Truth Aquatics at (805) 963-3564.

Camping
A limited number of primitive campsites are available on East Anacapa Island. From the landing dock, a steep stairway (154 steps) leads to the top of the bluff, and then it is a one-half mile walk to the campsites. Backpacking equipment is recommended for transporting food and camping gear. Pit toilets and picnic tables are provided; bring your own water, windbreak, and shelter. Stake your tent well; it gets very windy. Open fires are prohibited. For reservations and permits contact the National Park Reservation System (800) 365-CAMP.

Hazards

Turbulent seas and swift currents are common in the vicinity of Arch Rock. Avoid all areas of surging or breaking water. Dense fog is most common in June and July. Santa Ana winds can occur any time of the year but are most common from September to November. Wear a helmet and PFD, and carry a waterproof flashlight when exploring the caves. In an emergency, park rangers can be reached by radio on Channel 16.

Public access

Landing is permitted on East Anacapa Island beaches. Access above the beaches at East Anacapa Island is by way of the landing cove only. The waters on the north shore of East Anacapa down to a depth of 60 feet are designated as a "natural area." To remove any type of aquatic life in this area is prohibited. Landing is prohibited on offshore rocks and islets. This tour is located within the Channel Islands National Marine Sanctuary.

Kayak surfing

The Anacapa Islands are not noted for good surfing waves.

Launching

From the dock at Landing Cove on Anacapa, kayaks must be lowered 10-12 feet to the water with a hoist. Maximum capacity of the hoist is 300 pounds, and extra line should be brought along to rig a lifting bridle to attach your kayak to the hoist. It's best to load your kayak before lowering it to the water so you don't have to load a boat which is moving up and down with the surge. Launching a kayak with a hoist is a two- to three-person job. A steel

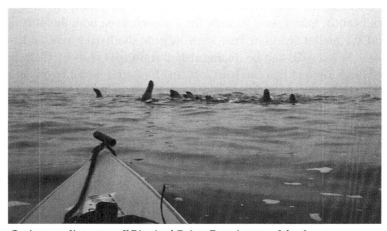

Curious sea lion pups off Pinniped Point, East Anacapa Island

ladder extends from the dock to the water. Negotiating the last step from the bottom of the ladder into your kayak can be difficult when there is a strong surge.

Tour description

From Landing Cove head toward the east end of the island. Western gulls, cormorants, brown pelicans, and red-billed oystercatchers swoop down from the towering bluffs as timid harbor seals quietly watch from a distance. The peaceful silence is occasionally interrupted by a loud blast from the foghorn located at the lighthouse high on the bluff overlooking the eastern end of the island. Directly ahead is Arch Rock, a well-known landmark with its 50-foot natural archway. The arch is separated from the east end of the island by a large, flat-topped rock. The currents are powerful and the water is turbulent as the swells surge between the menacing rocks. Passage through the archway should only be attempted during calm conditions.

The waters are rich with nutrients and the marine life is abundant. More than 27 species of cetaceans (whales and porpoises) visit the islands throughout the year. Whales are classified in two main groups, baleen whales and toothed whales. The most common baleen whales sighted at the islands are California gray whales, usually seen from December through March. Other baleen whales that can be seen are fin whales, blue whales, humpback whales, and minke whales. Toothed whales that sometimes visit the islands include the killer whale and the pilot whale.

The bluffs on the south side of the island are high and steep and the kelp beds hug the shore. The south side of Anacapa is somewhat protected from the predominant northwest swell, but it is exposed to southerly swells, common during the summer and fall. Pinniped Point is about three-quarter mile southwest of Arch Rock. A total of five species of pinnipeds live on the Channel Islands. Eared seals include the California sea lion, the northern fur seal, and the Steller sea lion. True seals include the harbor seal and the elephant seal. Eared seals can be distinguished from true seals by their external ears and hind flippers that can turn forward for better mobility on land. True seals lack external ears and, since they cannot turn their hind flipper, are only able to wiggle on their bellies on land. The loud barking of the California sea lions can be heard from nearly a half-mile. Hundreds of sea lions can be seen sunning themselves on the narrow beach to the east of Pinniped Point. Always remain a safe distance offshore to avoid disturbing the animals. Marine mammals are protected by both federal and state laws that interpret any action that modifies their behavior as harassment.

Return to Landing Cove following the same route.

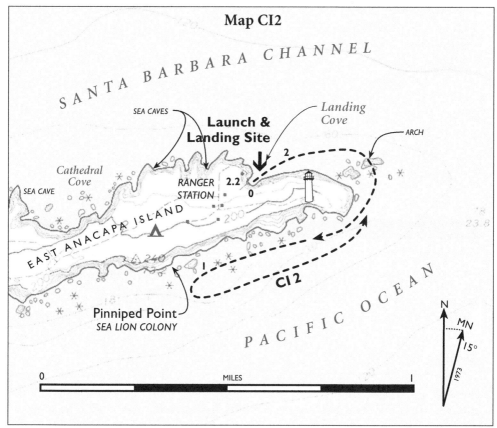

Tour CI2: East Anacapa Island—Landing Cove to Pinniped Point

Landing

Land at the dock at Landing Cove. To Hoist your kayak from the water to the dock will require two people. From the water, one person attaches the bridle to the kayak while the other operates the hoist. Boats may not remain tied to the dock. Storage of kayaks on the dock should be coordinated with the park ranger.

What to do afterward

On a calm day, the water in Landing Cove is very clear, and good for swimming or snorkeling. The bluffs surrounding the cove are nearly vertical and the water drops off quickly to a depth of twenty to thirty feet. Always be alert for boats which may be entering the cove.

Alternate tour: VT1

For more information
Island Packers (805) 642-1393
Truth Aquatics (805) 963-3564
Channel Islands National Park Visitors Center (805) 658-5730;
    www.nips.gov/chis
Channel Islands National Marine Sanctuary (805) 966-7107

TOUR CI3 SANTA CRUZ ISLAND:
Scorpion Bay to Cavern Point

Tour Details

Skill level:	Beginner
Trip length/type:	3.5 miles; round-trip; open-ocean; two to three hours (depending on the number of caves you want to explore)
Chart/map:	NOAA Chart #18729; USGS *Santa Cruz Island-D* 7.5 min series

Summary
Bright orange garibaldi, purple sea urchins, lavender algae, golden sea stars, and red abalone are all included on this colorful kayak adventure at Santa Cruz Island. This trip is a perfect introduction to kayaking the Channel Islands.

How to get there
Santa Cruz Island is located approximately 25 miles south of Santa Barbara Harbor. Daily excursions to Scorpion Bay at Santa Cruz Island are available year-round through Island Packers or Truth Aquatics, authorized concessionaires to the Channel Island National Park. For information and reservations, call Island Packers at (805) 642-1393 or Truth Aquatics at (805) 963-3564

Camping
A limited number of primitive campsites are available at Scorpion Bay. There is no pier (one is planned for the future), so campers are brought ashore in a skiff. Be prepared to get wet. Campers must transport their gear about one-half mile from the beach to the campsite. Pit toilets and picnic tables are provided; water is not. Campfires are permitted and firewood is available. For reservations and permits contact National Park Reservation System (800) 365-CAMP.

Hazards

Scorpion Bay is on the northeast end of Santa Cruz and is somewhat sheltered from the prevailing westerly and northwesterly wind and waves. Dense fog is most common in June and July. Santa Ana winds can occur any time of the year but are most common from September to November. Wear a helmet and PFD, and carry a waterproof flashlight when exploring the caves. In an emergency, park rangers can be reached by radio on Channel 16.

Public access

The eastern end of the Santa Cruz Island is owned by Channel Islands National Park. Private non-commercial kayakers may land on any eastern Santa Cruz Island beach and hike the interior without a permit. For the most recent information regarding permits and regulations contact Channel Islands National Park. The western ninety percent of Santa Cruz Island is owned by the Nature Conservancy. For information call (805) 962-9111. Landing is prohibited on offshore rocks and islets. This tour is located within the Channel Islands National Marine Sanctuary.

Kayak surfing

Good surfing waves can be found on the southeast side of Santa Cruz Island.

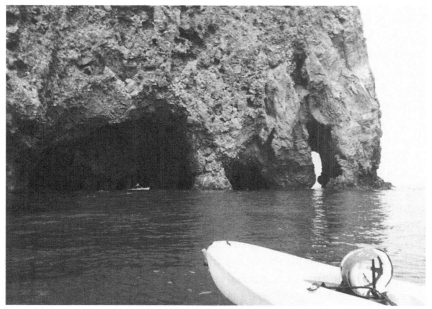

The jagged volcanic rocks are honeycombed with sea caves

Launching

Launch from the sand beach at Scorpion Bay. The waves are usually small and break near the shore, but a surf launch may be necessary.

Tour description

Santa Cruz Island is the largest and most environmentally diverse of the Channel Islands. Rugged mountains, deep valleys, year-round streams, and a diverse variety of plants and animals can all be found within the 96 square miles that encompass the island. The island is surrounded by 77 miles of pristine coastline with rocky cliffs, wide sandy beaches, offshore islands, colorful tide pools, and sea caves.

Chumash Indians inhabited the island for over 6000 years. As many as 2000 Indians at a time lived on the island, hunting, fishing and producing the "shell-bead money" which was used for trading with the mainland tribes. According to legend, the island was named "La Isla de Santa Cruz" (the island of the sacred cross) after a cross-tipped staff, which was accidentally left on the island by a priest from the Portola Expedition of 1769, was returned by a Chumash Indian.

Ranching activities began on Santa Cruz Island in 1839. Thousands of cattle and sheep once grazed the hillsides and the fertile valleys were planted with a variety of crops. Award-winning wines were produced on the island during the early 1900s. Remnants of the ranching era which can be seen today at Scorpion Bay include an historic adobe and several ranch buildings .

Scorpion Bay is located at the mouth of a large canyon on the northeast corner of the island. The bay is partially protected from the predominant northwesterly winds but is unprotected from Santa Ana winds. Occasionally during the late afternoon and evenings, strong offshore winds blow down Scorpion Canyon and out to sea.

From the beach at Scorpion Bay proceed northwest. The brown, volcanic cliffs are honeycombed with caves. Directly ahead at the base of the rocky headland are three sea caves. The cave on the left is the largest and passes through the point. Paddle through the cave, or if conditions are unfavorable, paddle around the point and continue heading northwest.

The precipitous bluff is over a hundred feet in height and drops straight into the sea offering no area for landing. Surging waves move rhythmically up and down the wall of rock revealing a variety of brightly-colored plants and animals clinging to the rough textured surface. The water is deep and the thick beds of giant kelp hug the shoreline. The cry of gulls and oystercatchers echoes through the air and pelicans flying in perfect formation skim along the wave tops. Around the next point is a relatively shallow cave with a portal over 100 feet high. The cobble beach at the back of the cave is occupied by several harbor seals peering out of the darkness with their wide, bulging eyes.

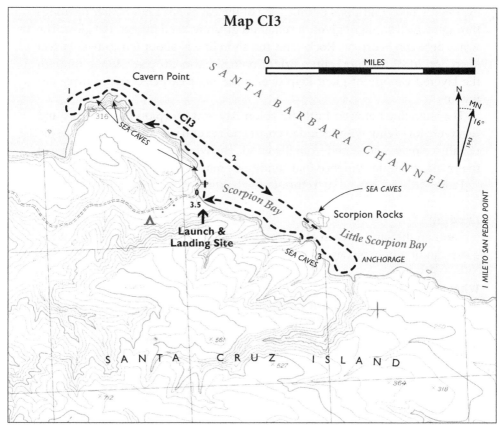

Map CI3

Tour CI3: Santa Cruz Island—Scorpion Bay to Cavern Point

Cavern Point, approximately one mile northwest of Scorpion Bay, is a major headland that shelters the northeast corner of the island from the prevailing wind. On the west side of the point is a large sea cave that extends to a depth of over 250 feet. Inside the cave the air is cool and damp. The dim light reveals slick, wet walls dripping with moisture. The sound of the surging waves echoes throughout the chamber.

From Cavern Point head back past Scorpion Bay to Little Scorpion Bay. A westerly tail wind should help give you a push along the way. Keep a lookout for dolphins which are commonly seen off the island during the summer and fall. California gray whales pass through the area during the winter and spring.

Little Scorpion Bay is a well-protected embayment just to the east of Scorpion Bay. Two large rocks (Scorpion Rocks), a short distance offshore, provide shelter for boats anchored to leeward. The rocks are nesting grounds for gulls and cormorants and landing is prohibited. Several sea caves can be explored when conditions permit. One of the caves has underwater openings through which sunlight gives the emerald green water a fluorescent glow. The water between Scorpion Rocks and the shoreline is about ten to twenty feet deep and ideal for snorkeling. Bright orange garibaldi pass slowly through the layered canopy of giant kelp over a sea floor carpeted with purple sea urchins.

The shoreline between Little Scorpion Bay and Scorpion Bay is rocky and relatively low-lying with secluded coves and several sea caves. Conditions are usually calm and sheltered from the wind. The wreck of a boat, deep in one of the caves, is ample evidence that conditions may not always be so placid.

From Little Scorpion Bay return to the landing at Scorpion Bay.

Landing

Land on the sandy beach at Scorpion Bay. Conditions are usually calm but a surf landing may be necessary.

What to do afterward

East Santa Cruz Island has several miles of self-guiding hiking trails. Trail guides are available from the park ranger. Fishing is permitted off the east end of the island, however no invertebrates may be taken form the shore.

Alternate tour: VT1

For more information

Island Packers (805) 642-1393
Truth Aquatics (805) 963-3564
Channel Islands National Park Visitors Center (805) 658-5730;
    www.nips.gov/chis
Channel Islands National Marine Sanctuary (805) 966-7107

TOUR CI4 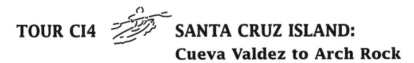 SANTA CRUZ ISLAND:
Cueva Valdez to Arch Rock

Tour Details

Skill level:	Intermediate.
Trip length/type:	4.7 miles; round-trip; open-ocean; two to three hours (depending on the number of caves you want to explore)
Chart/map:	NOAA Chart #18728; USGS *Santa Cruz Island-B* 7.5 min series

Summary

Located near the northwest corner of Santa Cruz Island, Cueva Valdez is seldom visited by kayakers. A large cave with a sea and land entrance provides access to a beautiful cove with a year-round stream. Sea caves, natural arches, abundant wildlife, and solitude are all included in the Cueva Valdez adventure.

How to get there

Cueva Valdez is located on Santa Cruz Island, approximately 25 miles south of Santa Barbara Harbor. Cueva Valdez is accessible by private boat or by special arrangement with the Island Packers or Truth Aquatics, authorized concessionaires to the Channel Island National Park. Daily excursions to

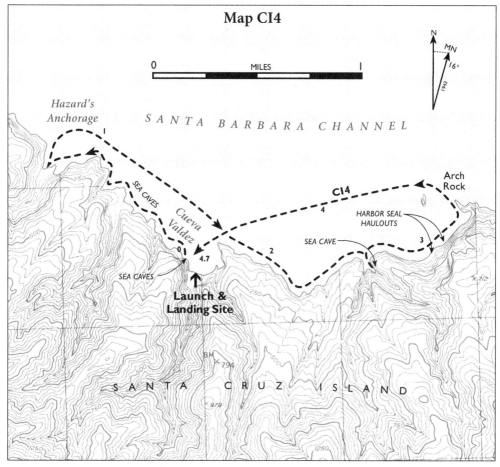

Tour CI4: Santa Cruz Island—Cueva Valdez to Arch Rock

Scorpion Bay, located at the east end of the island, are available year-round through the concessionaires. For information and reservations, call Island Packers at (805) 642-1393 or Truth Aquatics at (805) 963-3564.

Camping

For information on camping on the west end of Santa Cruz Island, call the Nature Conservancy at (805) 962-9111.

Hazards

The northern shore of Santa Cruz Island is exposed to the prevailing winds and waves, making conditions unpredictable and often rough. Watch for shallow submerged reefs in the vicinity of Arch Rock. Dense fog is most common in June and July. Santa Ana winds can occur any time of the year but are most common from September to November. Wear a helmet and PFD, and carry a waterproof flashlight when exploring the caves. In an emergency, park rangers can be reached by radio on Channel 16.

Public access

The western ninety percent of Santa Cruz Island is private land owned by the Nature Conservancy. A permit, which can take 10-12 days to process, is required to land. To obtain a landing permit, contact the Nature Conservancy at (805) 962-9111. Landing is prohibited on offshore rocks and islets. This tour is located within the Channel Islands National Marine Sanctuary.

Kayak surfing

The northwestern shore of Santa Cruz Island is not noted for good surfing waves.

Launching

Launch from the large cave on the west side of the cove at Cueva Valdez. An exit from the back of the cave leads to the sandy beach. The sea is usually calm but a surf launch may be necessary.

Tour description

Cueva Valdez is one of few sheltered coves on the northwest shore of Santa Cruz Island. During the summer and fall, boaters from Santa Barbara Harbor often visit this isolated anchorage. I was fortunate enough to get a ride with some friends of mine on their beautiful sailboat.

From Cueva Valdez cove, head northwest past a couple of rocky headlands that drop steeply to the water. If conditions are calm paddle close to the bluff face and observe the sea life clinging to the rocks. Just ahead is a large sea cave. The gentle gurgling of moving water echoes from within. Inside the cave the air is damp and cool. As you drift slowly ahead, the sunlight quickly fades. Your headlamp reveals a wide chamber with a high ceiling. The damp walls are covered with a lavender algae. To the left the cave narrows and the silence is broken by a startling roar as fine mist bellows from a blow hole in the rock. Extinguish the headlamp. As your eyes adjust to the darkness, notice the water is illuminated by light coming through a submerged opening to the cave. Exit the sea cave following the same route.

Hazard's Anchorage is located at the mouth of a narrow canyon about three-quarters of a mile northwest of Cueva Valdez. A wide sandy beach provides for an easy landing during calm conditions. The secluded beach is a perfect place to relax and enjoy the solitude and tranquility of Santa Cruz Island. Painted Cave, one of the largest known sea caves in the world, is about one and one-half miles northwest of Hazard's Anchorage. The cave is nearly one-quarter mile long and 100 feet wide. During the spring, a waterfall flows over the entrance. The Painted Cave is not included in this tour because sea conditions were unfavorable at the time of my visit.

From Hazard's Anchorage head back past Cueva Valdez. Arch Rock is the prominent point about one and three-quarter miles northeast of Cueva Valdez. Between Cueva Valdez and Arch Rock the bluffs are low-lying and the terrain slopes more gradually toward the coast. There are several large sea caves and narrow cobble beaches but this area is very exposed to the prevailing wind and waves. The secluded cobble beaches are a favorite haul-out for harbor seals and sea lions.

About one mile east of Cueva Valdez is a small cove at the mouth of a steep canyon. Within the cove is a cave that is dry at low tide and easy to explore. During the winter and spring a waterfall flows over the entrance to the cave.

At Arch Rock, towering natural archway extends through the headland. Observe conditions carefully before paddling though the arch; the currents can be powerful and the seas treacherous.

From Arch Rock, return to Cueva Valdez.

Landing

Land in the large cave at the west side of the cove at Cueva Valdez. An exit from the cave leads to the sandy beach. The waves are usually small and break near the shore but a surf landing may be necessary.

What to do afterward

Cueva Valdez is a beautiful cove to explore. There are several caves and at the east end of the cove is a small stream. Scuba diving and snorkeling are excellent. A permit is required to land.

Alternate tour: CI3

For more information
  Island Packers (805) 642-1393
  Truth Aquatics (805) 963-3564
  Nature Conservancy at (805) 962-9111
  Channel Islands National Park Visitors Center (805) 658-5730;
      www.nips.gov/chis
  Channel Islands National Marine Sanctuary (805) 966-7107

TOUR CI5   SANTA ROSA ISLAND:
Ford Point to Johnson's Lee

Tour Details

Skill level:	Intermediate.
Trip length/type:	4.0 miles; one-way; open-ocean; two to three hours
Chart/map:	NOAA Chart #18727, 18728; USGS *Santa Rosa Island-South* 7.5 min series

Summary
   How does camping on a secluded beach on one of the most beautiful islands on the California coast sound? Try the south side of Santa Rosa Island.

How to get there
   Santa Rosa Island is located approximately 32 miles southwest of Santa Barbara Harbor. Tour CI5 is located on the south side of Santa Rosa Island and is accessible only by private boat or by special arrangement with the Island Packers or Truth Aquatics, authorized concessionaires to the Channel Island National Park. Transportation to Beecher's Bay, on the northeast corner of Santa Rosa Island, is available year-round through the concessionaires. For information and reservations, call Island Packers at (805) 642-1393, Truth Aquatics at (805) 963-3564 or Channel Islands Aviation (Santa Rosa Island only) (805) 987-1301.

Camping
   Camping is permitted at the Water Canyon campground at Beecher's Bay. Campers must carry their gear one and one-half miles over flat ground from the landing pier to the campground. Picnic tables, wind breaks, water and pit toilets are provided. This is the only campground (in the Channel Islands

National Park) that has fresh water available. Beach camping is permitted at three-quarters of the beaches around the island. All beaches are subject to seasonal closures. For information on beach camping only, contact the Channel Islands National Park Visitor Center (805) 658-5730. For all other camping information, reservations and permits contact the National Park Reservation System (800) 365-CAMP.

Hazards

The south side of Santa Rosa Island is protected from the prevailing northwesterly wind and waves and conditions can be relatively calm even when 40-knot winds are blowing on the north side of the island. As on all the Channel Islands however, conditions are extremely unpredictable, so be prepared for the possibility of high winds and large waves. South swells that commonly occur during the summer months can create hazardous launching or landing conditions. Strong offshore winds frequently blow off the island in the late afternoon and evening. Dense fog is most common in June and July. In an emergency, park rangers can be reached by radio on Channel 16.

Public access

Without a permit, kayakers may land at Santa Rosa Island beaches for day use only. Certain beaches are subject to seasonal closures. Landing is

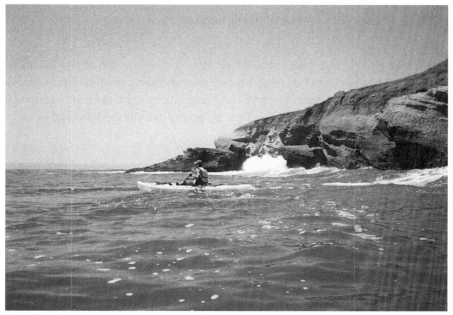

Strong south swells can create hazardous conditions for launching or landing on the South side of Santa Rosa Island

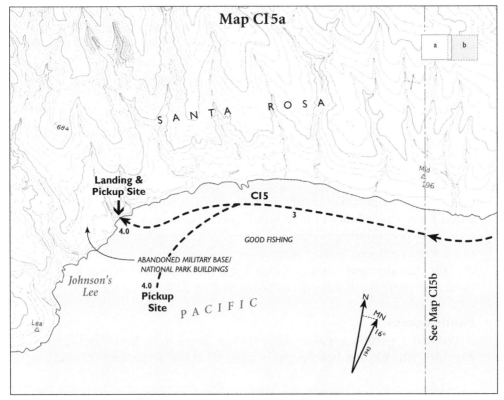

Tour CI5: Santa Rosa Island—Ford Point to Johnson's Lee

prohibited on offshore rocks and islets. Hiking the interior of the island is allowed without a permit or ranger escort except during the fall. For the most recent information regarding permits and regulations contact Channel Islands National Park Visitor Center. This tour is located within the Channel Islands National Marine Sanctuary.

Kayak surfing

During the summer and fall, swells generated from South Pacific storms can generate good waves on the headlands and beaches between Ford Point and Johnson's Lee.

Launching

The south side of Santa Rosa Island is protected from the prevailing northwesterly winds and swells. Conditions for launching are usually favorable but a surf launch may be necessary during a south swell. On this tour I was dropped off by the Island Packers in the water off Ford Point.

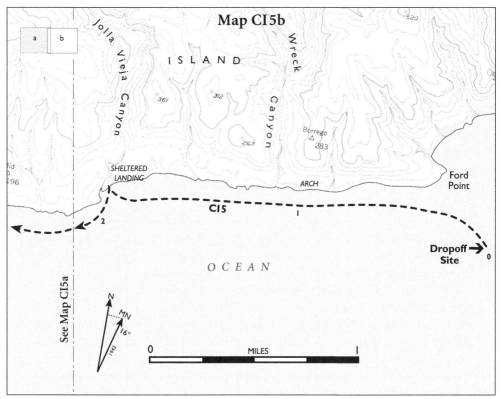

Tour CI5 (continued)

Tour description

From Ford Point follow the shoreline southwest. The white, sandy beach is long, narrow, and relatively straight with rocky headlands. Shallow caves and arches can be found on some of the headlands. The light-brown sandstone bluff varies in height and is backed by steeply sloping grassy hillsides. Occasional deep, narrow canyons lead to the water's edge. Landing sites are numerous and a surf landing is usually not necessary except during the fall when the waves are from the south.

Santa Rosa Island, the second largest of the Channel Islands, is fifteen miles long and ten miles wide. Archeological sites with human remains dating back at least 10,000 years, and the remains of dwarf mammoths dating back at least 12,000 years have been found at several locations on the island. A drop in sea level during the Ice Age exposed the four northern Channel Islands as a large land mass. During the period of lower sea level, it is believed that dwarf mammoths may have swam across the narrow channel separating the off-shore land mass from the mainland. Subsequent melting of the ice caps at the end of the last Ice Age led to a rise in sea level, isolating the islands from the mainland.

Cattle can sometimes be seen grazing high above the ocean on the grassy hillsides. Since the middle 1800s Santa Rosa Island has been used for ranching purposes. Eighty-five percent of the island's eighty-four square miles are non-native grasslands introduced by ranching operations. Although the introduction of non-native plants and animals to the island has been damaging, fifteen rare or endangered plant species and three endemic species have survived. Two groves of native Torrey pine, which grow only on Santa Rosa Island and on the mainland near San Diego, are found near Beecher's Bay on the east side of the island. The Torrey pine is the rarest pine tree in the world with only about 6,000 trees remaining.

Water visibility is usually good and wildlife is abundant. Sea lions, harbor seals, California gray whales, fin whales, blue whales, dolphins, and porpoises can all be seen at various times of the year. During the summer and fall fishing for yellowtail, halibut, and white seabass is excellent .

The white, sandy beaches between Ford Point and Johnson's Lee are perfect for camping. During the summer and fall the winds are generally light and fog is unusual. Warm ocean currents keep the water temperature a few degrees warmer than on the northern side of the island. During south swells, good waves can be found on the south-facing beaches. Santa Rosa is currently the only island on which beach camping is allowed. A permit is required and some beaches are restricted at certain times of the year to allow for animal breeding. Check with the park ranger for closures and restrictions.

Johnson's Lee is probably the most sheltered anchorage (from a northwesterly wind) on Santa Rosa Island. When the wind is gusting to 40 knots on the north side of the Santa Rosa Island, Johnson's Lee can be flat calm. Several small pocket beaches east of the point are easily accessible. Yachts and fishing boats frequently anchor offshore. Several roads and the remnants of a former military installation can be seen on the hillside. Most of the buildings have been removed and the facility has been converted to a park ranger station. Beware of the remains of an old decaying pier on the beach in front of the ranger station.

Landing

Conditions at Johnson's lee are usually calm but a surf landing may be necessary during a south swell. On this tour I was picked up by the Island Packers in the water off Johnson's Lee.

What to do afterward

Several miles of hiking trails are accessible from the Water Canyon campground at Beecher's Bay.

Alternate tour: VT1

For more information
Island Packers (805) 642-1393
Truth Aquatics (805) 963-3564
Channel Islands National Park Visitors Center (805) 658-5730; www.nps.gov/chis
Channel Islands National Marine Sanctuary (805) 966-7107

TOUR CI6 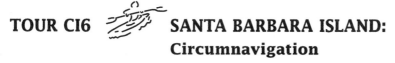 SANTA BARBARA ISLAND: Circumnavigation

Tour Details	
Skill level:	Intermediate
Trip length/type:	6.0 miles; round-trip; open-ocean; three to four hours
Chart/map:	NOAA Chart #18756; USGS *Santa Barbara Island* 7.5 min series

Summary
Once called Santa Barbara Rock, this square mile of craggy, volcanic rock surrounded by vertical cliffs hundreds of feet high, appears as if it had just been thrust from the seafloor. A new adventure awaits you around each point on your circumnavigation of this remote Channel Island.

How to get there
Santa Barbara Island is located approximately 46 miles southwest of Los Angeles. Transportation to Landing Cove at Santa Barbara Island is available through Island Packers or Truth Aquatics, authorized concessionaires to the Channel Island National Park. For information and reservations, call Island Packers at (805) 642-1393 or Truth Aquatics (805) 963-3564.

Camping
A limited number of primitive campsites are available on Santa Barbara Island. From the landing dock, a trail leads to the top of the bluff and then it is a short distance to the campsites. Backpacking equipment is recommended for transporting food and camping gear. Pit toilets and picnic tables are provided; water, windbreaks, and shade are not. Stake your tent well; it gets very windy. Open fires are prohibited. For reservations and permits contact National Park Reservation System (800) 365-CAMP.

Hazards

Because Santa Barbara Island is small and exposed, there are no all-weather landing sites. Most of the island is surrounded by vertical cliffs with few beaches to land on during an emergency. Plan your tour for the morning to avoid the strong afternoon westerly winds. Dense fog is most common in June and July. Santa Ana winds can occur any time of the year but are most common from September to November. Wear a helmet and PFD, and carry a waterproof flashlight when exploring the caves. In an emergency, park rangers can be reached by radio on Channel 16.

Public access

A permit is not required to land on Santa Barbara Island. However access to the island is allowed only at the landing cove. The waters on the east shore of Santa Barbara are closed to invertebrate fishing in waters less than 20 feet deep. Landing is prohibited on offshore rocks and islets. For the most recent information regarding permits and regulations contact Channel Islands National Park Visitor Center. This tour is located within the Channel Islands National Marine Sanctuary.

Kayak surfing

Santa Barbara Island is not noted for good surfing waves.

Launching

Launching from the dock at Landing Cove on Santa Barbara Island is a two- to three-person job. Kayaks must be lowered 10-12 feet to the water and there is not a hoist. It's best to stow your gear in your kayak before lowering it to the water so you don't have to load a boat which is moving up and down. A steel ladder extends from the dock to the water. Negotiating the last step from the bottom of the ladder into your kayak can be difficult when there is a large surge. A launch can also be made from the shore adjacent to the dock, but the rocks are sharp and the surge is strong. A strong south swell can make launching extremely dangerous.

Tour description

Only about one square mile in size, Santa Barbara Island is the smallest of the Channel Islands. The island is triangular in shape with high precipitous cliffs on all sides. Two prominent peaks protrude above the marine terrace. Signal Peak, at 635 feet, is the highest point on the island. Because of a lack of fresh water and overgrazing during past ranching activities, the island is only sparsely vegetated. The most prominent native plants are the giant coreopsis, a species of sunflower, and the prickly pear cactus. During the spring the fields of bright yellow flowering coreopsis give the island a golden glow. Most

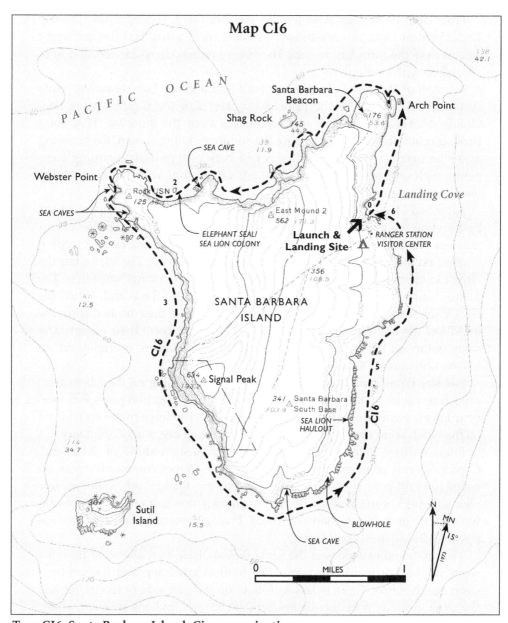

Map CI6

PACIFIC OCEAN

Santa Barbara Beacon

Shag Rock

Arch Point

SEA CAVE

Webster Point

Rock USN

SEA CAVES

East Mound 2

Landing Cove

ELEPHANT SEAL/ SEA LION COLONY

Launch & Landing Site

RANGER STATION VISITOR CENTER

SANTA BARBARA ISLAND

Signal Peak

Santa Barbara South Base

SEA LION HAULOUT

Sutil Island

BLOWHOLE

SEA CAVE

0   MILES   1

Tour CI6: Santa Barbara Island: Circumnavigation

of the island is covered with non-native grasses introduced by agricultural
activities during the 1920s.

Head north from the landing cove to Arch Point. If conditions permit, paddle beneath the arch. A navigational beacon atop Arch Point flashes every 5
seconds.

From Arch Point head west toward Webster Point, staying inside of Shag Rock. Vertical cliffs of dark-brown volcanic rock nearly 500 feet in height ascend from the turbulent waters. The craggy rock is sharp, jagged, and honeycombed with caves.

Just east of Webster Point are elephant seal and sea lion rookeries. Santa Barbara Island is one of the principal rookeries of the California sea lion. Hundreds of sea lions can be seen hauled out along the shoreline. Their loud barking echoes off the cliffs. During the summer mating season, the breeding males become very territorial. Males will bark continuously, warning competing males to stay clear. Confrontations often occur with fights involving intense pushing and biting.

After San Miguel Island, Santa Barbara is the second most important sea bird nesting site in the Channel Islands. The western gull, three species of cormorants, the brown pelican, and the black storm petrel (the rarest breeding sea bird on the California coast) all nest on the steep cliffs. The island has the largest known breeding colony in the world of the rare Xantus' murrelets. The Xantus' murrelets nest on the steep cliffs surrounding the island. When the chicks are only 48 hours old, they instinctively leave their nests during the middle of the night and fall to the ocean where they meet their parents and swim out to sea to spend the rest of their lives. The Xantus' murrelets return to land only during the nesting season.

Webster Point is probably the most spectacular setting on the island with numerous caves, arches, and offshore rocks. Curious sea lion pups surround your kayak, swimming and playing in the water. The huge males hauled out on the beach seem uninterested, provided everyone keeps a safe distance.

From Webster Point head south along the western shore of the island. Conditions can be rough during the afternoon. Waves commonly break on submerged offshore rocks and the kelp beds are thick. Sutil Island, a huge rock with high, vertical cliffs, lies approximately one-half mile off the southwest corner of the Santa Barbara Island. Passage between the two islands is possible during most conditions.

The south and east sides of the Santa Barbara Island are sheltered from the westerly and northwesterly wind. The bluff is low-lying and backed by a steep, sandy slope. There is less kelp than on the east side of the island and the water visibility is frequently greater than 50 feet. Sea lions are everywhere: in the caves, on the rocks, in the water, even climbing hundreds of feet up the steep hillsides. Young pups body surf in the waves just inches from the sharp rocks. Near the southwest corner of the island a giant blow hole spouts a geyser of water up to 20 feet into the air.

Head north along the east side of the island to Landing Cove. The wind often blows offshore and the sea is calm in the lee of the bluff. The landing cove is a great place for snorkeling. The water is very clear and usually calm.

The sea lions that hang out in the cove are accustomed people and are very friendly.

Landing

Land at the dock where you launched. Hoisting a kayak from the water to the dock is a job best accomplished by two people. Boats may not remain tied to the dock. Storage of kayaks on the dock should be coordinated with the park ranger. A landing can also be made onto the shore adjacent to the dock, but the rocks are sharp and the surge is strong. A strong south swell can make landing extremely dangerous.

What to do afterward

Santa Barbara Island has a small visitor center with displays and six miles of hiking trails. A trail guide is available at the visitor center. Due to the fragile environment, hiking is limited to the well-marked trails and collecting of cultural and natural resources is prohibited.

Alternate tour: VT1

For more information

Island Packers: (805) 642-1393

Truth Aquatics (805) 963-3564

Channel Islands National Park Visitor Center at (805) 658-5730;
www.nps.gov/chis

Channel Islands National Marine Sanctuary (805) 966-7107

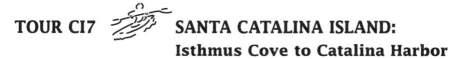

TOUR CI7　SANTA CATALINA ISLAND:
Isthmus Cove to Catalina Harbor

Tour Details

Skill level:	Advanced
Trip length/type:	17.5 miles (18.0 with portage to Isthmus Cove); round-trip; open-ocean; six to seven hours
Chart/map:	NOAA Chart #18757; USGS *Santa Catalina Island-North* and *Santa Catalina Island-West* 7.5 min series

Summary

You're not likely to pass many other kayakers on this trip around Santa Catalina's rugged and remote west end. Play with the frisky sea lions off Gull

Rock, experience the roaring blowhole in Iron Bound Bay, and explore the history of Catalina Harbor.

How to get there
Santa Catalina Island is located about 20 miles southwest of San Pedro. Daily excursions to Avalon and Two Harbors (Isthmus Cove) are available year-round through several concessionaires. For information, call the Avalon Chamber of Commerce and Visitor Center at (310) 510-1520.

Camping
Developed campgrounds are available at Two Harbors, Parson's Landing, Avalon, and Little Harbor. Primitive camping is also available. Rental kayaks are available at Two Harbors and Avalon. For information, reservations, and permits contact Two Harbors Visitor Services at (310) 510-2800

Hazards
Stiff headwinds are likely during the afternoon between Lion Head and the west end. Confused seas, thick kelp beds, and strong currents may be encountered at the west end of the island, and along the southwest side of the island all the way to Ribbon Rock. A south swell may cause hazardous seas on the south side of the island. Beware of Whale Rock, a shallow, submerged rock about one mile southeast of Ribbon Rock. Dense fog may be encountered almost any time of the year.

Public access
Eighty percent of Santa Catalina Island is owned by the Nature Conservancy. Without a permit, kayakers may land at Catalina beaches for day use only. Certain beaches may be subject to seasonal closures. A permit is required for back-country travel beyond the beach. For the most recent information regarding permits and regulations, contact the Santa Catalina Island Conservancy (310) 510-1421.

Kayak surfing
The west end of Catalina Island is not noted for good surfing waves.

Launching
Launch from the beach at Isthmus Cove. A surf launch is seldom necessary.

Tour description
Santa Catalina Island is the most populous of the Channel Islands with about 2,200 permanent residents. During the summer, the population swells as thousands of boaters and tourists from around the world visit the "Magic

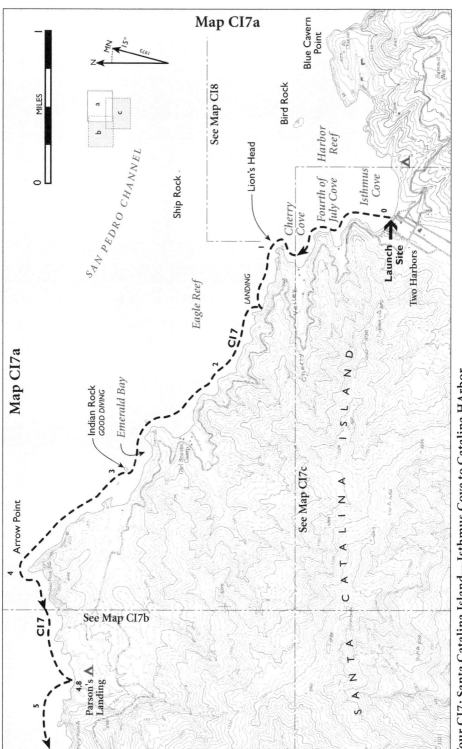

Map CI7a

Tour CI7: Santa Catalina Island—Isthmus Cove to Catalina HArbor

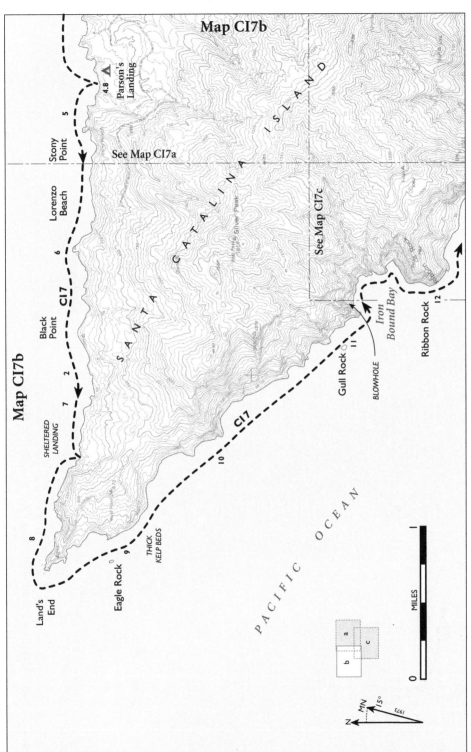

Map CI7b

Parson's Landing

4.8

5

Stony Point

See Map CI7a

Lorenzo Beach

6

CI7

Black Point

2

7

SHELTERED LANDING

8

Land's End

9

Eagle Rock

THICK KELP BEDS

10

CI7

SANTA CATALINA ISLAND

West Peak Silver Peak

Iron Bound Bay

See Map CI7c

12

Ribbon Rock

11

Gull Rock

BLOWHOLE

PACIFIC OCEAN

Map CI7b

MN 15°

1973

N

MILES

1   0

a

b

c

Tour CI7 (continued)

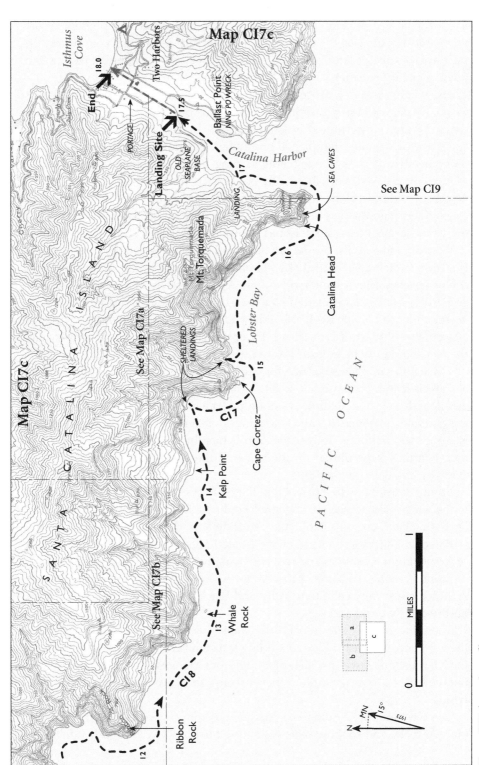

Map CI7c

Isthmus Cove

Two Harbors

Ballast Point
NING PO WRECK

End 18.0

PORTAGE

17.5

Landing Site

OLD SEAPLANE BASE

Catalina Harbor

17

LANDING

SEA CAVES

See Map CI9

SANTA CATALINA ISLAND

See Map CI7a

Mt. Torquemada

16

Catalina Head

SHELTERED LANDINGS

Lobster Bay

15

CI7

Cape Cortez

14

Kelp Point

PACIFIC OCEAN

See Map CI7b

13

Whale Rock

CI8

Ribbon Rock

12

Map CI7c

MILES

0

a

c

b

N

MN

15°

1973

Tour CI7 (continued)

Isle." The city of Avalon, at the eastern end of the island, is a popular resort where most of the island's residents live. Two Harbors, a small community on the narrow strip of land between Isthmus Cove and Catalina Harbor, is the other population center.

From Isthmus Cove proceed north past Fourth of July Cove and Cherry Cove. During summer, hundreds of pleasure boats moor in the sheltered coves. Landing is permitted in Isthmus Cove, but Fourth of July and Cherry coves are private and landing is prohibited. Separating the coves are sheer, rocky headlands backed by steeply sloping hillsides vegetated with coastal sage, chaparral, scrub brush, prickly pear cactus, and grasses. California ironwood, an endemic plant found on the north facing slopes of the island, was once widespread on the California mainland. A grove of Catalina cherry trees, one of the largest trees on the island, grows in the valley behind Cherry Cove.

West of Lion Head, a prominent headland on the west side of Cherry Cove, is a long stretch of beautiful shoreline. Several small coves with gravel and cobble beaches offer a sheltered landing. Approximately one mile offshore lies Ship Rock, a tall guano-covered rock that, from a distance, appears like a large vessel under sail. Eagle Reef, a shallow reef extending well offshore, lies about one mile northwest of Lion Head. Except during large northwesterly swells the reef should not be a hazard to kayakers.

Three miles northwest of Isthmus Cove is Emerald Bay, noted for its emerald green water. Indian Rock, a small island in the middle of the bay, offers excellent diving. The shallow waters support a wide variety of sea life including garibaldi, sheephead, calico bass, rays, lobster, and scallops. Emerald Bay is a popular anchorage for boaters and is bustling with activity during summer. Landing is permitted on the beach at the east end of the cove. Please abide by all posted regulations.

From Emerald Bay to Arrow Point the bluffs are very high and drop steeply to the water's edge with no sheltered landings. During the afternoon, strong headwinds and currents can make paddling very difficult.

Parson's Landing is a sandy cove located about two-thirds of a mile west of Arrow Point. Campers and tents are usually visible on the beach.

From Parson's Landing, proceed to the west past Stony Point. Several secluded coves between Stony Point and Black Point offer some shelter from northwesterly wind and seas.

The wind usually stiffens and the waves become larger as you approach the west end. The last sheltered landing is a small cove below a low saddle in the island about three-quarters of a mile from the west end. If conditions are unfavorable for passage around the west end, this cove can provide a suitable refuge.

The west end of Catalina is a narrow, precipitous point of land with submerged rocks and shallow reefs extending offshore. On the south side of the headland about 300 yards offshore is Eagle Rock. Passage between Eagle Rock and the island is possible under most conditions. Thick kelp beds extend well offshore and paddling can be difficult. The southwest side of the island is steep, rugged, and sparsely vegetated. The beach is narrow and rocky with few suitable landing spots. During summer, south swells pound the unprotected shoreline, churning up the sediment and giving the water a milky green color.

From Eagle Rock head for Ribbon Rock, which lies about three miles southeast. The first sheltered landing site on the south side of the island is Iron Bound Bay, which is just northwest of Ribbon Rock. Gull Rock, which lies just offshore, is a favorite sea lion haul-out. Iron Bound Bay is a well-defined anchorage with high vertical bluffs. The water in the bay is deep and visibility good. A large blow hole on the northwest side of the bay interrupts the tranquil setting with a repetitious roar and an explosive fountain of spray.

Ribbon Rock is a dark-faced, rocky palisade with thick bands of white quartz rock that look like raveled spools of ribbon. A variety of sea birds nest on the rocky ledges high above the turbulent water. Two-thirds of a mile past Ribbon Rock is Whale Rock, a large, submerged rock about fifty yards offshore. Large waves can build up quickly around Whale Rock, so be sure to give it plenty of room. In the lee of Whale Rock is a broad bay offering some protection from a west or northwest swell but no protection from a south swell. At the east end of the bay is a cobble beach offering a suitable location for landing under most conditions. The beach is littered with driftwood, crab and lobster traps, and foam fishing floats.

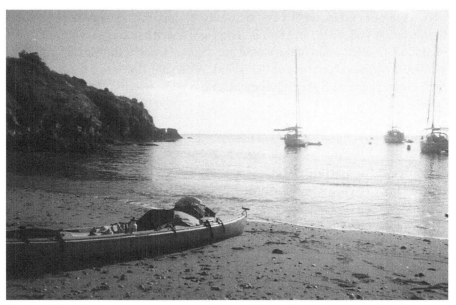

Howland's Landing is a protected cove to the east of Emerald Bay, Santa Catalina Island

Cape Cortez is a very picturesque point, with beautifully sculptured rocks and crystal-clear water. On the east side of the point is a long, narrow cove with a sandy beach that is well protected from west and northwest weather and seas. To the east of Cape Cortez is Lobster Bay, another wide bay offering good protection from northwesterly wind and waves. South swells pound the bay, activating several spectacular blow holes. Commercial divers harvest sea urchins from the bay.

Catalina Head, a prominent point of land, separates Lobster Bay from Catalina Harbor. The craggy headland is honeycombed with sea caves. On the lee side of the point is Catalina Harbor, the most sheltered anchorage on the entire island. Catalina Harbor has been used as the setting for several movies, including the original *Mutiny on the Bounty* with Clark Gable. During World War II the US Navy used the harbor as a seaplane base. The remains of the old seaplane pier can still be seen. Rotting timbers of the *Ning Po*, a Chinese junk built in China in 1773, lie in the mud inside Ballast Point. Today there are two private-yacht-club facilities in the harbor and numerous boat moorings.

Landing

Land at the floating dock at the north end of Catalina harbor. Restrooms and picnic facilities are provided. If returning to Isthmus Cove, a portage is necessary across the relatively level, one-half-mile strip of land separating the two harbors.

What to do afterward

Two Harbors offers lots to do, including hiking, biking, snorkeling, scuba diving, beach volleyball, and tennis. There is a snack bar and a restaurant with great food. Guided tours of the island are available, and a shuttle bus provides transportation to other parts of the island. A general store stocks marine supplies, fishing gear, camping equipment, and a wide selection of food and beverages.

Alternate tour: CI8

For more information

Two Harbors Visitor Services (310) 510-1550
Avalon Chamber of Commerce and Visitors Bureau (310) 510-1520;
  www.catalina.com
Catalina (Two Harbors) Harbor Department (310) 510-2683
Avalon Harbor Department (310) 510-0535
Santa Catalina Island Conservancy (310) 510-1421;
  www.catalinas.net/seer/demomenu.htm

TOUR CI8 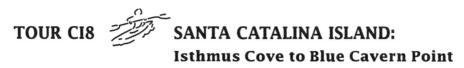 SANTA CATALINA ISLAND:
Isthmus Cove to Blue Cavern Point

Tour Details	
Skill level:	Beginner
Trip length/type:	4.8 miles; round-trip; open-ocean; two to three hours
Chart/map:	NOAA Chart #18757; USGS *Santa Catalina Island-North* 7.5 min series

Summary
Spectacular sea caves and clear blue water await you on this short, easy tour, perfect for the beginner paddler.

How to get there
Santa Catalina Island is located about 20 miles southwest of San Pedro. Daily excursions to Avalon and Two Harbors (Isthmus Cove) are available year-round through several concessionaires. For information, call the Avalon Chamber of Commerce and Visitor Center at (310) 510-1520.

Camping
Camping is available at Two Harbors (Isthmus Cove), Parson's Landing, Avalon, Little Harbor, and several other locations on the island. Picnic tables, fire pits, barbecues, and chemical toilets are provided. Most campgrounds have water and showers. Rental kayaks are available at Two Harbors and Avalon. For information, reservations, and permits contact Two Harbors Visitor Services at (310) 510-2800.

Hazards
Confused seas and gusty winds are likely during the late afternoon off Isthmus Cove. Headwinds are likely to be encountered when returning from Blue Cavern Point to Isthmus Cove. Santa Ana winds and dense fog can be encountered almost any time of the year.

Public access
Eighty percent of Santa Catalina Island is owned by the Nature Conservancy. Without a permit, kayakers may land at Catalina beaches for day use only. Certain beaches may be subject to seasonal closures. A permit is required for back-country travel beyond the beach. For the most recent information

regarding permits and regulations, contact the Santa Catalina Island Conservancy (310) 510-1421.

Kayak surfing

The north side of Catalina Island is not noted for good surfing waves.

Launching

Launch from the beach at Isthmus Cove. A surf launch is rarely necessary.

Tour description

From Isthmus Cove proceed northeast to Little Fisherman Cove. Two Harbors Campground and a private-yacht-club facility are located on the beach; private yachts lie at anchor offshore. About two-thirds mile northeast of Isthmus Cove is Big Fisherman Cove, home of the University of Southern California's Marine Laboratory. Landing in the cove is prohibited.

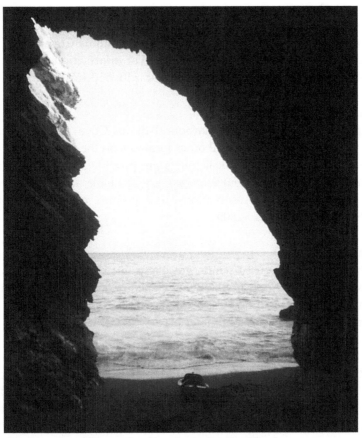

Sea Cave west of Parsons Landing, Santa Catalina Island

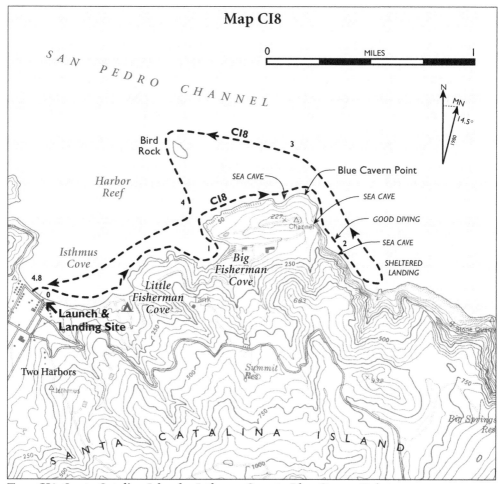

Map CI8

Tour CI8: Santa Catalina Island—Isthmus Cove to Blue Cavern Point

The shoreline and near-shore waters from Big Fisherman Cove to Blue Cavern Point are protected as a nature preserve and collecting sea life or artifacts is prohibited. Steep cliffs of solidified volcanic ash drop straight into the sea. At Blue Cavern Point is the largest of several sea caves in the area. The cave is about 200 feet in length and extends from one side of the point to the other. A short distance east of the point is a small beach where conditions are generally favorable for landing. Good diving is easily accessible from the beach.

The water off Blue Cavern Point is deep and exceptionally clear. A vertical rock wall with underwater caves and cornices drops from sea level to a depth of about 50 feet. A variety of fish, including the garibaldi, sheephead, kelp bass, opaleye, and perch, can be seen feeding along the rocky ledges. Sheephead, rather unusual fish, are born females and change to males late in life. Males have a deep-blue-to-black head and tail, a white lower jaw, and a pinkish mid section. Females are usually a reddish color, with a much more rounded head. They have large buck teeth which they use to crush their prey.

Schools of jack mackerel glistening in the sunlight swim in perfect precision through the long, flowing strands of kelp. Occasionally a yellowtail tuna or barracuda appears from nowhere seeking unwary prey. Horn sharks, moray eels, and lobster hide in the dark shadows while giant bat rays lie motionless on the sandy bottom.

From Blue Cavern Point head to Bird Rock, a low-lying white rock several hundred yards offshore. The island is covered in bird guano and landing is not recommended but the diving is good. A shallow reef extends northwest and west of the island. Harbor Reef lies about one-quarter mile southwest of Bird Rock. From Bird Rock return to Big Fisherman Cove and follow the shoreline back to Isthmus Cove. A strong headwind and choppy seas may be encountered during the afternoon.

Landing

Land on the beach at Isthmus Cove where you launched. A surf landing is rarely necessary.

What to do afterward

Two Harbors offers lots to do, including hiking, biking, snorkeling, scuba diving, beach volleyball and tennis. There is a snack bar and a restaurant with great food. Guided tours of the island are available and a shuttle bus provides transportation to other parts of the island. A general store stocks marine supplies, fishing gear, camping equipment, and a wide selection of food and beverages.

Alternate tour: CI9

For more information

Two Harbors Visitor Services (310) 510-1550
Avalon Chamber of Commerce and Visitors Bureau (310) 510-1520;
        www.catalina.com
Catalina (Two Harbors) Harbor Department (310) 510-2683
Avalon Harbor Department (310) 510-0535
Santa Catalina Island Conservancy (310) 510-1421;
        www.catalinas.net/seer/demomenu.htm

TOUR CI9 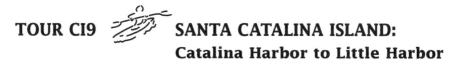 SANTA CATALINA ISLAND:
Catalina Harbor to Little Harbor

Tour Details	
Skill level:	Intermediate
Trip length/type:	9.7 miles; round-trip; open-ocean; three to four hours
Chart/map:	NOAA Chart #18757; USGS *Santa Catalina Island-West* and *Santa Catalina Island-North* 7.5 min series

Summary

Little has changed on this remote part of the island since the Gabrielino Indians paddled these waters in their wooden-planked canoes.

How to get there

Santa Catalina Island is located about 20 miles southwest of San Pedro. Daily excursions to Avalon and Two Harbors (Isthmus Cove) are available year-round through several concessionaires. For information, call the Avalon Chamber of Commerce and Visitor Center at (310) 510-1520.

Camping

Camping is available at Two Harbors (Isthmus Cove), Parson's Landing, Avalon, Little Harbor, and several other locations on the island. Picnic tables, fire pits, barbecues, and chemical toilets are provided. Most campgrounds have water and showers. Rental kayaks are available at Two Harbors and Avalon. For information, reservations, and permits contact Two Harbors Visitor Services at (310) 510-2800.

Hazards

Choppy and unsettled conditions are likely during the afternoon. Westerly winds blow directly on-shore and waves are reflected off the steep bluffs between Catalina Harbor and Little Harbor. A shallow reef extends off the entrance to Little Harbor. Watch for submerged rocks when entering the harbor. Landing or launching on the south side of the island may be impeded by a southerly swell. Dense fog may be encountered almost any time of the year.

Public access

Eighty percent of Santa Catalina Island is owned by the Nature Conservancy. Without a permit, kayakers may land at Catalina beaches for day use only. Certain beaches may be subject to seasonal closures. A permit is

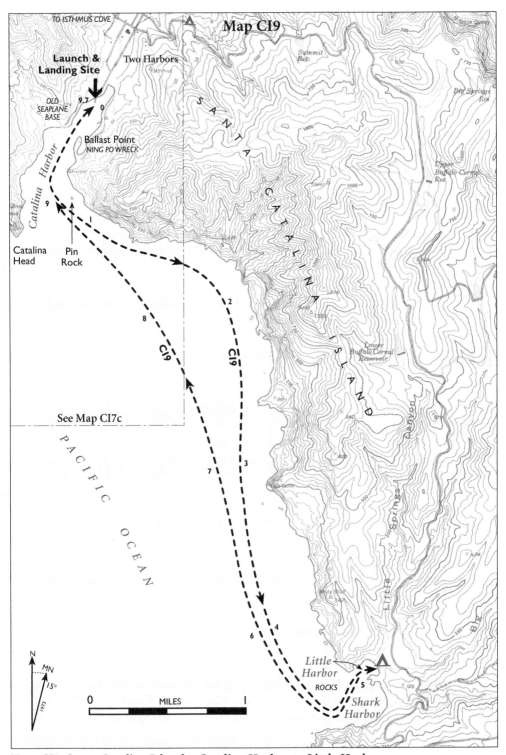

Tour CI9: Santa Catalina Island—Catalina Harbor to Little Harbor

required for back-country travel beyond the beach. For the most recent information regarding permits and regulations, contact the Santa Catalina Island Conservancy (310) 510-1421.

Kayak surfing

Waves for kayak surfing can be found at Shark Harbor, and at Ben Weston Beach (not included in this tour) about one-mile south of Little Harbor.

Launching

Launch from the floating dock at the north end of Catalina harbor. Restrooms and picnic facilities are provided. If coming from the Isthmus Cove, a portage is necessary across the relatively level, one-half-mile strip of land separating the two harbors.

Tour description

From Catalina Harbor follow the coastline to the southeast. On a clear day, the most distant visible point of land southeast is China Point. Little Harbor is about half way between Catalina Harbor and China Point. This part of Catalina Island is desolate and sparsely vegetated. Landslides are common. Steep, talus slopes extend to the water's edge and the beaches are narrow and discontinuous.

During calm conditions, landing is possible in several of the coves along this route. The beaches are remote and accessible only by boat. When the waves are big, beach sediment is churned up, giving the water a milky green color.

Little Harbor is an excellent landing site, protected by a natural rocky shoal extending off the point on the north side of the cove. The shoal is a series of exposed rocks and shallow reefs. Enter the bay to the south of the shoal. A small headland separates Little Harbor from Shark Harbor. Large waves, which can be good for surfing, sometimes break in Shark Harbor.

Archeological excavations at Little Harbor indicate human habitation dating back over 4,000 years. Several groups of native inhabitants probably occupied the area over time. The most recent inhabitants were the Gabrielino Indians, who arrived about 500 B.C. The Gabrielinos were closely related to the Indians of the Los Angeles area and the southern Channel Islands. They mostly lived off the sea, hunting and fishing from their seaworthy canoes. Their peaceful life was disrupted first by the Spanish missionaries and later by the Russian and Yankee fur traders who arrived in the early 1800s. By 1832 the last of the Gabrielinos were removed from the island to be resettled on the mainland. Today the only remains of the original inhabitants of the island are the piles of shell and bone called middens which can be seen on the bluffs overlooking the cove at Little Harbor.

One of the most beautiful campgrounds on the island is located at Little Harbor. The campsites are spacious and furnished with picnic tables, fire pits, barbecues, community toilets, and showers. A shuttle-bus service is available for transportation to Avalon, the Airport in the Sky, and Two Harbors.

From Little Harbor, return to Catalina Harbor following the same route. A headwind can be encountered during the afternoon.

Landing

Land from the floating dock at the north end of Catalina harbor. Restrooms and picnic facilities are provided. If returning to Isthmus Cove, a portage is necessary across the relatively level, one-half-mile strip of land separating the two harbors.

What to do afterward

A walk through Two Harbors provides a glimpse of its long and colorful history. In 1863 hundreds of miners swarmed to Catalina Island in search of gold and silver. In 1864 the US Army sent troops to the isthmus to take control of the island from the miners. The barracks built to house the soldiers and the commanding officer's quarters still stand today and can be seen on the road between Isthmus Cove and Catalina Harbor. On the hillside overlooking Two Harbors is the Banning House, built in 1910 by the Banning Brothers,

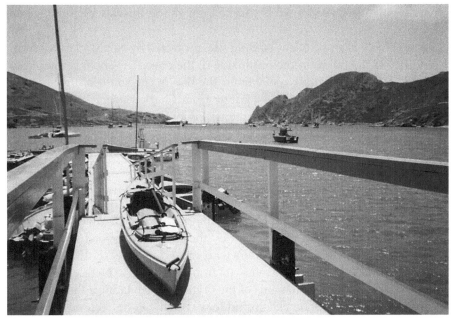

Boat dock at Catalina Harbor, Santa Catalina Island

then the owners of the island. The house has been renovated and today serves as a bed and breakfast inn.

Alternate tour: CI8

For more information
    Two Harbors Visitor Services (310) 510-1550
    Avalon Chamber of Commerce and Visitors Bureau (310) 510-1520;
        www.catalina.com
    Catalina (Two Harbors) Harbor Department (310) 510-2683
    Avalon Harbor Department (310) 510-0535
    Santa Catalina Island Conservancy (310) 510-1421;
        www.catalinas.net/seer/demomenu.htm

Ventura County Tours

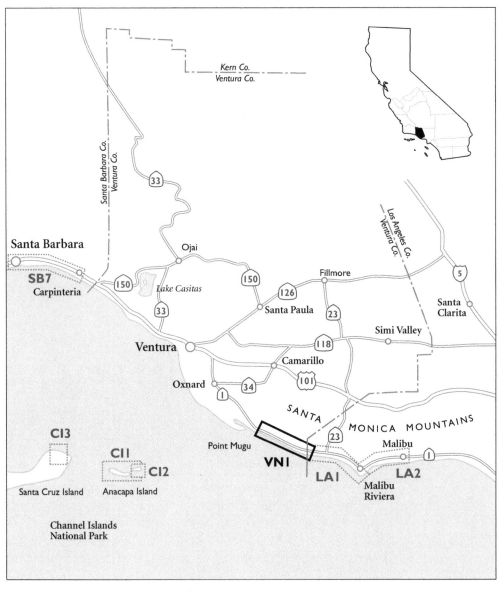

Tour	Skill Level	Length
VN1: Point Mugu to Leo Carillo State Beach	Intermediate	8.2 miles

Chapter 6

Ventura County

The band of orange sky narrowed and was replaced with deep purples and reds as the sun sank beneath the horizon. The familiar silhouettes of Anacapa and Santa Cruz islands stood out clearly against the fading light. A short distance offshore, a brightly lit fishing boat moved slowly back and forth in search of its elusive prey. The air was beginning to cool but the sand was still warm from the afternoon sun. It had been a long day and we were very relaxed as we sat in our beach chairs reminiscing over the day's events.

Our adventure had begun that morning at Point Mugu Beach. The strong Santa Ana wind, that had blown for most of the previous night, finally subsided leaving behind a smooth, flat sea. We paddled close to Mugu Rock and then headed east along Thornhill Broome Beach. The sky was hazy and the ocean a subtle blue-gray. The hills were parched and dry after seven months without rain. It was already quite warm and we were ready for a swim by the time we stopped at Sycamore Cove for a lunch break.

After lunch and a stroll around the picturesque cove, we were back on the water. The air was dead calm and the sea was smooth as glass. It was one of those rare fall days that you never forget. As I settled into a rhythmic stroke, I imagined what it must have been like hundreds and even thousands of years ago when the Chumash Indians paddled their tomol canoes across these same waters. Not much had changed except the busy highway that hugged the shoreline.

By mid afternoon we had reached County Line, a spot that I used to surf when I was growing up. The waves were small, but as usual there were a few die hard surfers scrapping for the infrequent waves. A short distance beyond, we explored some offshore rocks. The water was clear and the colorful seafloor was illuminated by the penetrating rays of the afternoon sun.

We landed on the north side of Sequit Point at Leo Carillo State Park, and set up our tents at the paddle camp, an area on the beach set aside for kayakers to camp for the night. There was still plenty of daylight so we went for a short hike in the hills overlooking the campground. It felt good to stretch our legs and the panoramic view of the coastline was spectacular.

I was tired and it was getting late. The silhouetted islands had melted into the darkness leaving only the flashing beacon from the lighthouse on East Anacapa. A gentle breeze, scented with the sweet smell of sage, drifted off the land. Except for the occasional wave washing up on the beach, the night was still as I crawled into my warm sleeping bag.

— *Leo Carillo State Beach, November 9, 1996*

TOUR VN1 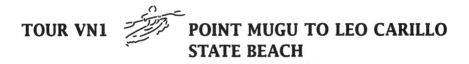 POINT MUGU TO LEO CARILLO STATE BEACH

Tour Details	
Skill level:	Intermediate
Trip length/type:	8.2 miles; one-way; open-ocean; three to four hours
Chart/map:	NOAA Chart #18740; USGS *Point Mugu* and *Triunfo Pass* 7.5 min series

Summary

Experience the past as you paddle this eight-mile stretch of rugged coastline. For thousands of years the Chumash Indians hunted and fished these waters from their wood planked canoes called *tomols*.

How to get there

To reach the launch site, exit Highway 1 at Point Mugu Beach just west of Mugu Rock. Parking, portable toilets, seasonal lifeguard services, and telephones are provided. Fee.

To reach the landing site, exit Highway 1 at Leo Carillo State Beach. Parking, restrooms, picnic facilities, seasonal lifeguard services, and telephones are provided. Fee.

Camping

Camping is available at Thornhill Broome Beach, La Jolla Valley, and Sycamore Canyon, all within Point Mugu State Park, and at Leo Carillo State Beach. Paddle Camps, dedicated to use by kayakers, are provided at the Thornhill Broome Beach and at North Beach in Leo Carillo State Beach. The Paddle Camps are a feature of the Lower Tomol Trail, an ocean-paddling trail dedicated in 1996. The trail extends from Point Mugu to the Santa Monica Pier. For information on the paddling trail, contact the Santa Monica Trails Council, P.O. Box 345, Agoura, CA 91301 or Point Mugu State Park. For camping reservations, call ParkNet (800) 444-7275.

Hazards

The water is very deep just a short distance offshore, and the waves emerge rather suddenly and sometimes without warning. The sandy beaches slope steeply at the water's edge, and the shore break and rip currents can be very strong. During large surf conditions all headlands and offshore rocks should

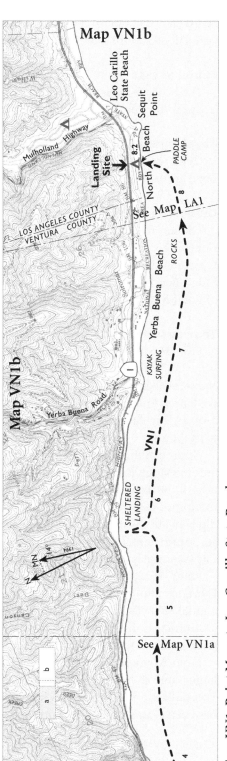

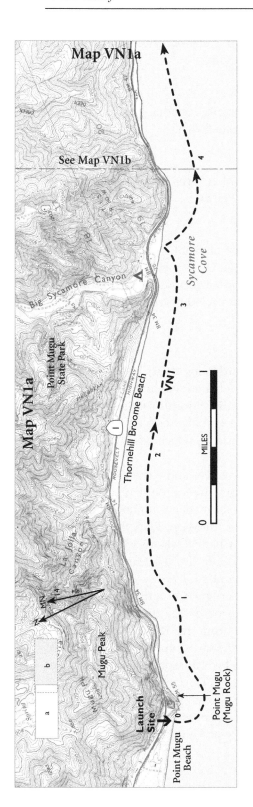

Tour VN1: Point Mugu to Leo Carrillo State Beach

be given a wide berth. Strong Santa Ana winds can occur at any time of the year. Always be prepared for the possibility of fog.

Public access

The beach is accessible to the public at Thornhill Broome Beach, Sycamore Cove, Yerba Buena Beach, and Leo Carillo State Beach.

Kayak surfing

Good waves for kayak surfing can be found at Yerba Buena Beach (County Line) and at Leo Carillo State Beach (Sequit Point).

Launching

Launch from Point Mugu Beach just west of Point Mugu. The shoreline slopes steeply and the waves and currents can be very strong. A surf launch is frequently necessary. If conditions are too hazardous to launch at Point Mugu Beach, launch from one of the more protected beaches on the east side of Point Mugu.

Tour description

From Point Mugu Beach, paddle east toward Point Mugu. To the northwest is the US Navy Pacific Missile Test Center. Contained within the Naval Center is the 1,800-acre Mugu Lagoon, one of southern California's largest remaining wetlands. Anacapa and Santa Cruz Islands are usually visible to the west. On a very clear day you can see Santa Barbara Island, which lies about 40 miles to the south.

Approach the Point Mugu cautiously; the waves and currents can be hazardous. Mugu Rock is the west end of the Santa Monica Mountains, which are part of the Transverse Mountain Ranges, the only major mountain ranges in California that trend in an east-west direction. At Mugu Rock the mountains dip beneath the ocean emerging again as the Channel Islands which are located approximately 16 miles to the west. Offshore lies the Mugu Submarine Canyon, nearly one-half mile deep and nine miles long.

Point Mugu is a good location for observing California gray whales. February and March are the best months for observing the whales on their annual 10,000-mile, round-trip migration from the Bering Sea to Baja California. California sea lions, harbor seals, and dolphins are commonly seen, as well a wide variety of sea birds. Kelp beds are sparse along this route.

From Mugu Rock continue southeast along Thornhill Broome Beach. A large sand dune is visible on the hillside behind the beach. In the past, Thornhill Broome Beach was known as "tin can beach," but today the beach has been cleaned up and incorporated into Point Mugu State Park.

The name Mugu came from the Chumash Indian word Muwu, which meant "beach." The Chumash lived in small villages along this part of the coast for nearly 7,000 years. They were hunters and fishermen who lived in large, dome-shaped houses with thatched roofs that housed up to four families. The Chumash built wood-plank canoes called *tomols* which they used for transportation up and down the coast and to the offshore islands. The wood for the canoes was carefully selected, then shaped and trimmed using sharp pieces of bone and shell. Holes were drilled in the planks using rock drills. The planks were then laid edge to edge and bound together with red milkweed fiber string. The outside of the *tomol* was sealed and painted with a mixture of tar, pine pitch, and red ochre color, then decorated with colorful abalone shells. A *tomol* was up to 30 feet in length and could hold up to 12 people.

The Chumash were an industrious people with a complex and highly structured society. They enjoyed storytelling, music, and games. According to one legend the first Chumash lived on Santa Cruz Island. They were created by the Earth Goddess Hutash from the seeds of a magic plant. The island became overcrowded, and the noise of all the people kept Hutash awake at night, so she decided that some of the people must move to the mainland. She made a very long rainbow bridge that stretched across the channel and directed her people to cross over the ocean on it but not to look down. Those who looked down, fell from the sky and were turned into dolphins to keep from drowning. For that reason, the Chumash considered dolphins their brothers and never hunted them.

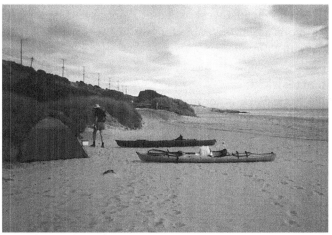

The "paddle camp" at Leo Carillo State Beach is part of the Lower Tomol Trail, an ocean paddling trail dedicated in 1996

Beyond Thornhill Broome Beach is Sycamore Cove, the location of the ranger headquarters for Point Mugu State Park. Parking, restrooms, telephones, and picnic facilities are available. The cove is sheltered and suitable for landing during most of the year. Behind the cove is Sycamore Canyon, a woodland with tall sycamore trees. An ancient Chumash village was located at the mouth of the canyon. The Boney Mountain Wilderness, in Sycamore Canyon, has several miles of scenic trails. The hillsides above Sycamore Canyon are vegetated with chaparral, California sage, and a variety of coastal scrub. The open slopes have only a few trees due to the fierce wildfires that periodically rage across the Santa Monica Mountains.

East of Sycamore Cove is a small headland from which you can see Point Dume, the Palos Verdes Peninsula, and Santa Catalina Island on a very clear day. Around the point is another long, narrow, sandy beach. The beach is accessible from Highway 1, and there are several suitable landing spots. At the east end of the beach is a popular surfing spot known as County Line. The waves have good shape and break on a north or south swell. The site is frequented by many surfers, so if you decide to ride some waves on your kayak, be polite; a kayak weighs a lot more than a surfboard.

East of the surf spot is a large group of white condominiums and homes overlooking the water. Several partly submerged rocks lie just offshore. If conditions are calm, paddle between the rocks and observe the colorful plants and animals in the clear, shallow water. Watch carefully for breaking waves, which can sometimes arrive unexpectedly. Leo Carillo State Beach is approximately one mile east of the condominiums.

Landing

Land at North Beach, just west of Sequit Point. A surf landing may be necessary. If conditions are unfavorable for landing at North Beach, try the cove in the lee of Sequit Point.

What to do afterward

Leo Carillo State Park is located at the mouth of Arroyo Sequit Creek, which was the site of a Chumash village for over 6,000 years. The campground is shaded with large sycamore trees and there are several miles of scenic hiking trails in the hills overlooking the campground. The clear waters off Sequit Point are noted for good fishing and diving.

Alternate tour: LA3

For more information

Point Mugu State Park Headquarters (805) 986-8591

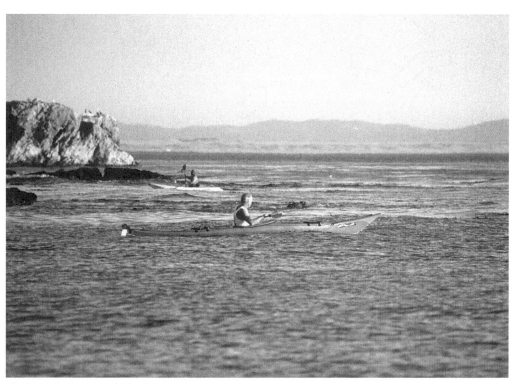

Shell Beach, San Luis Obispo County

Los Angeles County Tours

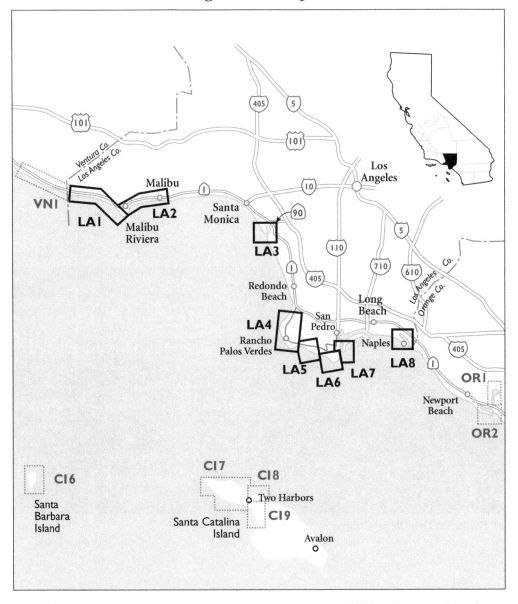

Tour		Skill Level	Length
LA1:	Leo Carillo State Beach to Westward Beach	Intermediate	8.5 miles
LA2:	Westward Beach to Malibu Pier	Intermediate	9.7 miles
LA3:	Marina del Rey	Beginner	4.7 miles
LA4:	Malaga Cove to Abalone Cove	Advanced	8.3 miles
LA5:	Abalone Cove to Royal Palms State Beach	Intermediate	4.5 miles
LA6:	Royal Palms State Beach to Cabrillo Beach	Beginner	2.7 miles
LA7:	Port of Los Angeles	Intermediate	6.5 miles
LA8:	Alamitos Bay	Beginner	5.5 miles

Chapter 7

Los Angeles County

As I prepared my kayak for launching, I reminisced with the lifeguard about the good-old days in the South Bay. We had both grown up in the Los Angeles area and had a few common friends. He said things were different now; more houses, more cars, and a lot more people. I slid my kayak into the smooth water and headed south toward the distinctive flat-topped point a short distance away. I had passed this point hundreds of times as a kid, but I had never seen it from this perspective. One of the neat things about kayaking is that you get to see things you can't see from the land.

The day was sunny but there was a crispness in the air; not unusual considering it was Thanksgiving Day. Other parts of the county were already covered with snow. In California we often take our beautiful warm weather for granted.

The sea was glassy and the seemingly endless horizon was broken only by the familiar outline of Catalina Island. A group of pelicans glided silently past, their wingtips barely skimming the smooth water.

Off the end of the point was a large, flat reef with tide pools of all sizes and shapes. I paddled around the perimeter of the reef looking for a place to enter one of the tide pools. I found a narrow channel, leading to one of the pools, where the water was surging in and out. I paddled into the channel and an incoming wave lifted me and my kayak over the rocks and into the tide pool. The clear shallow pool was filled with an endless variety of colorful marine creatures which I examined in great detail. Afterward, I paddled back to where I had entered and patiently waited for a surge of water to retrieve me from the tide pool. Exiting the pool was like going over a small waterfall and often when I attempt this type of maneuver I end up getting dumped, but this time I managed to stay dry.

As I worked my way around to the eastern side of the point, I noticed a sea cave. It appeared large enough for my kayak and I could see light coming from within. I watched for a while to make sure it was safe and then entered. I moved quickly through the 50-foot-long cave, and found myself in a beautiful cove on the other side of the point. I stopped to take some pictures when all of a sudden I heard a crashing sound behind me. Before I could turn around I was capsized by a large wave that came roaring through the cave. I was climbing back into my kayak, when another wave came crashing through the cave and dunked me a second time. I swam about gathering the gear that had been washed off the boat then climbed aboard and paddled, unharmed but thoroughly humbled, to the beach.

— Portuguese Point, November 28, 1996

TOUR LA1 LEO CARILLO STATE BEACH TO WESTWARD BEACH (POINT DUME COUNTY BEACH)

Tour Details

Skill level:	Intermediate
Trip length/type:	8.5 miles; one-way; open-ocean; three to four hours
Chart/map:	NOAA Chart #18740; USGS *Triunfo Pass* and *Point Dume* 7.5 min series

Summary

Enormous mansions resembling medieval castles overlook this magnificent stretch of coastline with high bluffs and narrow sandy beaches.

How to get there

To reach the launch site, exit Highway 1 at Leo Carillo State Beach. Parking, restrooms, picnic facilities, lifeguard services and telephones are available. Fee.

To reach the landing site, exit Highway 1 at the south end of Zuma Beach at Westward Beach Road. Drive to the end of the road (Point Dume County Beach) and park near the rock headland at end of the beach. Parking, restrooms, picnic facilities, lifeguard services, and telephones are available. The beach closes at dark. Fee.

Camping

Camping is available at Thornhill Broome Beach, La Jolla Valley, and Sycamore Canyon, all within Point Mugu State Park (see Tour VN1), and at Leo Carillo State Beach. Paddle Camps, dedicated to use by kayakers, are available at Thornhill Broome Beach and at North Beach in Leo Carillo State Beach. The Paddle Camps are a feature of the Lower Tomol Trail, an ocean-paddling trail dedicated in 1996. The trail extends from Point Mugu to the Santa Monica Pier. For information on the paddling trail, contact the Santa Monica Trails Council, P.O. Box 345, Agoura, CA 91301 or Point Mugu State Park. For camping reservations, call ParkNet (800) 444-7275.

Hazards

The water is very deep just a short distance offshore, and the waves emerge rather quickly and sometimes without warning. The sandy beaches slope steeply at the water's edge, and the shore break and rip currents can be very strong. Zuma Beach and Westward Beach can be the most dangerous. During large wave conditions all headlands and offshore rocks should be given a wide berth. Strong Santa Ana winds can occur at any time of the year. Always be prepared for the possibility of fog.

Public access

Public access to the shoreline is available through the Robert H. Meyer Memorial State Beaches which include El Pescador, La Piedra and El Matador State Beaches. Parking at the state beaches is located on the bluff top, making access to the beach with a kayak difficult.

Kayak surfing

Good waves for kayak surfing can be found at Sequit Point.

Launching

Launch at North Beach, just west of Sequit Point. A surf launch may be necessary. If conditions are unfavorable, a more sheltered launch site may be found in the cove to the east of Sequit Point.

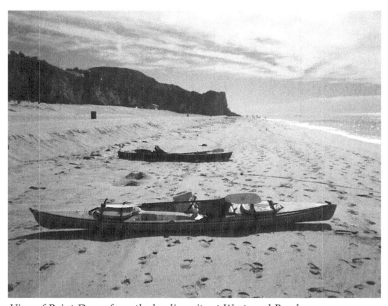

View of Point Dume from the landing site at Westward Beach

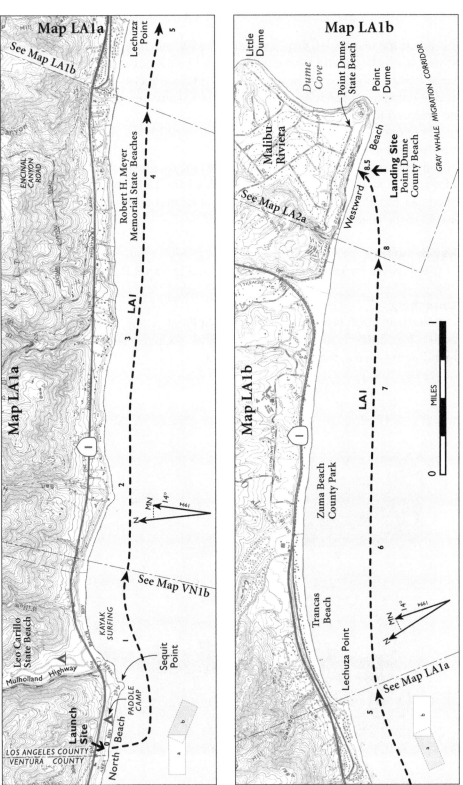

Map LA1a

See Map LA1b

Lechuza Point

Canyon

ENCINAL CANYON ROAD

Robert H. Meyer Memorial State Beaches

LA1

5

4

3

See Map VN1b

MN 14°
1994
N

2

Leo Carillo State Beach

Mulholland Highway

KAYAK SURFING

Sequit Point

PADDLE CAMP

1

Launch Site

North Beach

LOS ANGELES COUNTY
VENTURA COUNTY

a

b

Map LA1b

Little Dume

Malibu Riviera

Dume Cove

Point Dume State Beach

Point Dume

Westward Beach

Landing Site
Point Dume County Beach

8.5

8

See Map LA2a

GRAY WHALE MIGRATION CORRIDOR

Zuma Beach County Park

LA1

7

6

Trancas Beach

Lechuza Point

MN 14°
1994
N

0   MILES   1

See Map LA1a

5

a

b

Tour LA1: Leo Carillo State Beach to Westward Beach (Point Dume County Beach)

Tour description

Before embarking on your journey, spend some time exploring the tide pools and rock formations off Sequit Point. A variety of marine organisms including sea anenomes, sea slugs, urchins, mussels, limpets, and sea stars inhabit the rocky ledges. Offshore, garibaldi are frequently visible through the waving strands of giant kelp. Perhaps a pod of dolphins will ride the perfectly shaped waves that wrap around the rocky point.

Sequit Point was the site of a Chumash village for over 6,000 years. The word *Chumash* is derived from the word *michumash,* which had several meanings, one of which was "those who make shell bead money." The shell money was made of olivella and abalone shells of uniform size which were drilled using a chert drill and strung on sinew. The standard unit of measure was a string of shells wrapped once around the hand. The Chumash developed a vast network of trade that extended as far east as the Mojave Desert near the Colorado River.

From Sequit Point head east. On a clear day, Point Dume, about eight miles southeast, is visible. The coastline is relatively straight, with narrow, sandy beaches separated by occasional rocky headlands. The bluff is high and steep, with a narrow marine terrace. To the north the Santa Monica Mountains rise to an elevation of over 3,000 feet. Stately mansions, some resembling medieval castles, others appearing as abstract modern sculptures, overlook the sparkling blue ocean. Most of the bluff-top property is privately owned.

Approximately five miles east of Leo Carillo State Beach is Lechuza Point. To the east of the point is Trancas Beach, a residential community with numerous beach front homes. Catamaran sailboats can be seen on the beach in front of the homes. At Trancas Beach the coastline turns south and becomes more exposed to westerly winds and waves, making paddling often difficult during the afternoon. To the southeast is Zuma County Beach, the largest county-owned beach in Los Angeles. Facilities at Zuma Beach include parking, restrooms, picnic areas, and snack bars. Lifeguards are on duty year-round. Landing is not advisable at Zuma Beach due to the powerful waves and hazardous currents. Westward Beach is southeast of Zuma Beach on the west side of Point Dume.

Landing

Land about one-quarter mile northwest of Point Dume at Westward Beach. The waves can be strong and the currents powerful. A surf landing may be necessary. If conditions are unfavorable, a more suitable landing may be found at Corral State Beach on the east side of Point Dume.

What to do afterward

Westward Beach is a well-known location for whale watching. Between December and April, the giant mammals can be observed on their annual migration. March is probably the best month for whale watching, because the cow and calf pairs swim close to the beach to feed and relax in the warm, shallow water. At the southeast end of Westward Beach is Point Dume State Park, with hiking trails and tide pools. Fishing and diving are excellent off the point.

Alternate tour: LA3

For more information
Zuma Beach County Lifeguard Headquarters (310) 457-9891

TOUR LA2   WESTWARD BEACH (POINT DUME COUNTY BEACH) TO MALIBU PIER

Tour Details

Skill level:	Intermediate
Trip length/type:	9.7 miles; one-way; open-ocean; four to five hours
Chart/map:	NOAA Chart #18740, 18744; USGS *Point Dume* and *Malibu Beach* 7.5 min series

Summary
From the bold, windswept cliffs and the secluded coves of Point Dume to the glitter and fame of star-studded Malibu Colony, this tour offers something for just about everyone.

How to get there
To reach the landing site, exit Highway 1 at the south end of Zuma Beach at Westward Beach Road. Drive to the end of the road (Point Dume County Beach) and park near the rock headland at end of the beach. Parking, restrooms, picnic facilities, lifeguard services, and telephones are available. The beach closes at dark. Fee.

The landing site is on the west side of Malibu Pier. Malibu Pier is located at 23000 Highway 1 in Malibu. Park in the parking lot at Malibu Surfrider Beach (west of the pier) or on Highway 1 adjacent to the pier. The is also a small lot east of the pier. Restrooms, picnic facilities, lifeguard services, and telephones are available. Fee.

Camping

According to the trail guide for the Lower Tomol Trail (an ocean-paddle trail which was dedicated in 1996) arrangements can be made for kayakers to stay overnight at two hotels located on the beach at Malibu. The Tomol Trail extends from Point Mugu to the Santa Monica Pier. For information on the paddling trail and accommodations, contact the Santa Monica Trails Council, P.O. Box 345, Agoura, CA 91301 or Point Mugu State Park. Camping is available at Thornhill Broome Beach, La Jolla Valley, and Sycamore Canyon, all within Point Mugu State Park (see tour VN1), and at Leo Carillo State Beach. For reservations in the State Park campgrounds, call ParkNet (800) 444-7275.

Hazards

The wind, currents, and waves are generally more severe on the west side of Point Dume. The water is deep off Westward Beach and Point Dume causing waves to build up quickly and sometimes, to break without warning. Shallow submerged rocks extend over 200 yards off Point Dume. Strong Santa Ana winds can occur at any time of the year. Always be prepared for the possibility of fog.

Public access

Most of the coastal property between Point Dume and the Malibu Pier is privately owned. The best public access for kayaks is at Corral State Beach, which is located at the intersection of Corral Canyon Road and Highway 1. Seasonal lifeguard services are provided, and limited roadside parking is available along Highway 1.

Kayak surfing

Good waves for kayak surfing can be found at Point Dume, Little Dume Point, and Latigo Point. Malibu Surfrider Beach is for board surfing only.

Launching

Launch from Westward Beach. A surf launch may be necessary. If conditions are unfavorable for launching at Westward Beach, try Corral State Beach on the east side of Point Dume.

Tour description

Point Dume is a prominent headland that marks the northwest end of Santa Monica Bay and is visible for many miles up and down the coast. On a clear day, Santa Catalina Island, the Palos Verdes Peninsula, and the buildings of downtown Los Angeles are all visible from the point.

Several million years ago Point Dume was a volcanic island. Eventually the island was connected to the mainland by sand and silt deposited in the

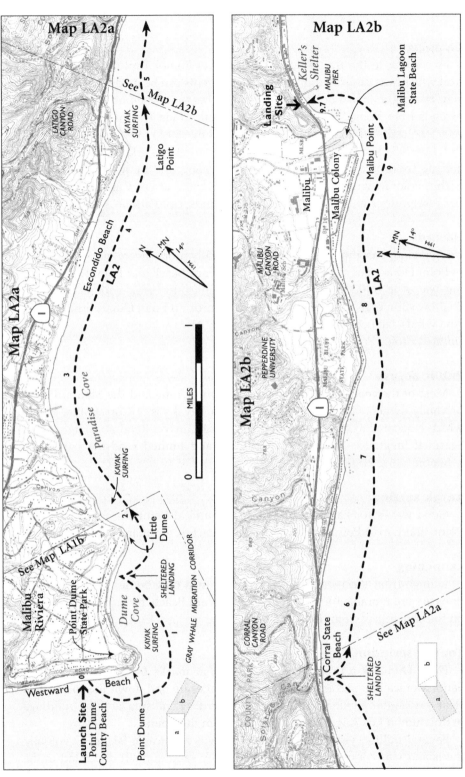

Tour LA2: Westward Beach (Point Dume County Beach) to Malibu Pier

shallow water between the two. Over millions of years the entire unit was uplifted by faulting and folding, creating the point we see today.

From Westward Beach paddle southeast toward Point Dume. Proceed cautiously when approaching the point. Partly submerged offshore rocks extend over 200 yards south of the point. Breaking waves and currents can be very hazardous. Due to the strong currents that sweep past the point, the water is remarkably clear and good for diving. Upwelling of cold, nutrient-rich waters from the Dume Submarine Canyon, which extends offshore, provide the perfect environment for a wide variety of sea life. Harbor seals, sea lions, and dolphins are commonly seen, and brown pelicans, cormorants, and gulls roost on the precipitous cliffs and the offshore rocks. Forests of giant kelp provide the habitat for a variety of rock fish. During winter and spring, Point Dume is an excellent location for viewing California gray whales.

On the east side of the point is Dume Cove, a relatively large embayment flanked by high, steep bluffs. Tide pools, on the west side of the cove, support a wide variety of colorful marine organisms. A narrow sand beach at the the foot of the bluff offers a suitable landing under most conditions. The only public access to Dume Cove is by a hiking trail from Windward Beach. "Little Dume" is a smaller point on the east end of the cove. Both Point Dume and Little Dume Point have good waves for kayak surfing.

Northeast of Little Dume the bluff top is privately owned and there is no public access to the beach. Beautiful homes perched precariously on the high bluff overlook the magnificent coastline. Approximately one and three-quarter miles northeast of Point Dume is Paradise Cove, a private beach. Facilities include a pier, restaurant, showers, restrooms, and picnic area. At Paradise Cove the coastline turns to the east forming a long, narrow, sandy beach known as Escondido Beach. Landing is favorable during most conditions, but access to the beach from Highway 1 is limited. At the east end of Escondido Beach is Latigo Point, a low rocky headland. Homes built on tall pilings are clustered along the water's edge. If you happen to be a structural engineer, this is a good place to study the different foundation designs for beach front homes. Several gaps in the continuous row of homes indicate that not all designs provide the same protection against the fury of the sea.

Latigo Point is a well known surf-spot. Perfectly shaped waves peel around the rocky point on either a west or a south swell. Because it is well known, the waves can be crowded when the "surf's up." Limited access is available from Latigo Road or from Corral State Beach, east of the point. Corral State Beach is a long, narrow, sand beach offering a favorable landing during most conditions. Roadside parking along Highway 1 is available as well as seasonal lifeguard services. Corral Beach is an alternative landing site if parking is unavailable at Malibu Pier.

East of Corral State Beach is the famous Malibu Colony. The beautiful homes of famous movie stars, musicians, and other celebrities line the shore. Which house is Johnny Carson's? Is it the tall gray mansion that looks like a fortress? Does Barbara Streisand live in the one painted a bright pink? Who owns the house that looks like a peacock's tail; was it the home that belonged to Sting?

At the east end of the Colony is a chain-link fence separating the rich and famous from the general public. Offshore are several large rocks marking the entrance to the Malibu Lagoon and the famous Malibu Surfrider Beach. As you head toward the pier, stay clear of the surfers; Surfrider Beach is for board surfing only.

Landing

Land on the sand beach just west of the Malibu Pier. Conditions are usually favorable, but a surf landing may be necessary during a south swell. Stay out of the surfing area.

What to do afterward

The Malibu Lagoon Museum is located at Malibu Lagoon State Park, west of the Malibu Pier. A variety of restaurants and shops are located within a short walking distance.

Alternate tour: LA3

For more information

Zuma Beach Lifeguard Headquarters (310) 457-9891

TOUR LA3   MARINA DEL REY

Tour Details

Skill level:	Beginner
Trip length/type:	4.7 miles; round-trip; marina; two to three hours
Chart/map:	NOAA Chart #18744; USGS *Venice* 7.5 min series

Summary

Marina del Rey is one of the world's largest and most modern small-craft harbors. Beautiful yachts, fine restaurants, shops, and grassy parks are all within easy reach on this relatively short and easy paddle.

How to get there

To reach the launch site exit the Marina Freeway (Highway 90) at Lincoln Boulevard and go right approximately one-half mile to Washington Boulevard. Go left on Washington to Via Marina, then left one block to Admiralty Way. Go left on Admiralty Way and then turn right immediately into Parking Lot 10. Telephones, restrooms, picnic facilities, and year-round lifeguard services are available. Fee.

Camping

Recreational vehicle facilities are available at Dockweiler RV Park, at the west end of Imperial Highway at Dockweiler Beach, about two and one-half miles south of Marina del Rey. For reservations, call ParkNet (800) 444-7275.

Hazards

This tour is entirely within Marina del Rey. Boat traffic can be congested; always follow the rules of the road. Avoid fishing lines when paddling near docks or jetties. Gusty winds and choppy conditions are likely near the harbor mouth during the afternoon. Fog can occur at any time of the year. If possible plan your trip route to have a following tidal current.

Public access

Public docks are located throughout the harbor.

Kayak surfing

Good waves for kayak surfing can be found on the beaches outside the breakwater at Marina del Rey.

Launching

Launch from the beach adjacent to the lifeguard tower at Mother's Beach. A surf launch is not necessary. Stay clear of designated swimming areas.

Tour description

Marina del Rey is the world's largest man-made recreational harbor. There are over 6000 yachts moored at the 17 privately owned anchorages and seven private yacht clubs. Boating facilities include marine supplies, hoists, and fuel docks. Bike paths, jogging paths, and walkways connect the four public parks within the harbor area. Shopping areas, restaurants, transient boat docks, and several hotels are all available within the one-and-one-third square mile area.

From Mother's Beach head east along Basin D toward the Main Channel. Turn right at the Main Channel and proceed south toward the harbor entrance. Stay on the right side of the Main Channel and watch for other boats when crossing A, B and C yacht basins, on your right. South of Basin A, the

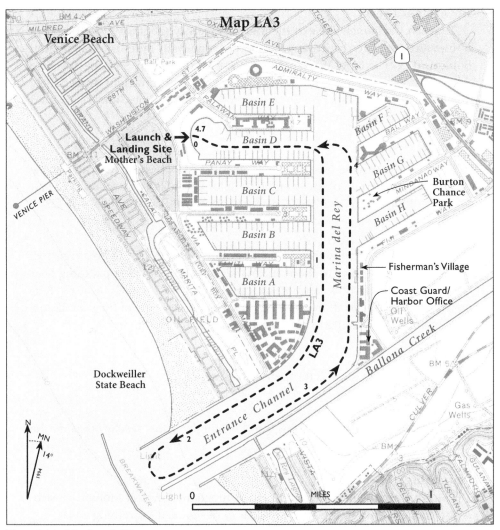

Tour LA3: Marina del Rey

Main Channel turns west, becoming the Entrance Channel. The north and south banks of the Entrance Channel are shielded by a rock jetty. Stay to the far right-hand side of the channel between the marker buoys and the rock jetty.

At the harbor mouth, cross to the south side of the Entrance Channel and proceed back into the harbor, staying to the right of the channel between the white buoys and the jetty. South of the jetty is Ballona Creek and the Ballona Wetlands. Prior to the development of Marina del Rey Harbor, the wetlands encompassed over 1,700 acres of marshlands and lagoons. Gabrielino Indians hunted and fished in the shallow marshlands. In the early 1900s, most of the lagoons were drained and Ballona Creek was channelized. In 1954 the Congress passed legislation authorizing dredging of the wetlands, and in 1960 construction of the harbor began. In 1962 the Marina del Rey Harbor opened. Today, only a few hundred acres of the once expansive wetlands remain. The Ballona Wetlands now provide one of the last remaining refuges in the area for migrating birds.

A public bike path along the top of the south jetty joins the South Bay Bicycle Trail, which extends approximately 20 miles from Torrance County Beach to Will Rogers State Beach.

At the UCLA Boathouse the channel turns north. On the right is the Harbor Master's office, Sheriff Station, Coast Guard Station, and Los Angeles County Lifeguard facility. Just north of the lifeguard facility is Fisherman's Village, a commercial replica of a New England Seaport with shops, galleries, restaurants, and recreational facilities. Kayak rentals are available at the guest dock.

Yacht Basins F, G and H are north of Fisherman's Village. Burton Chance Park, an eight-acre public park with restrooms, picnic facilities, walkways, and visitor docks is located between Basins G and H. After passing Basin G cross the Main Channel and enter Basin D. Mother's Beach is at the west end of Basin D.

Landing

Land on the sand beach adjacent to the lifeguard tower. Avoid the designated swimming areas.

What to do afterward

Bike riding, windsurfing, sailing, fishing, and beautiful beaches are all available in Marina del Rey. Tourist attractions such as Hollywood, Universal Studios, and the Getty Museum are all within a half-hour drive (if you're lucky).

Alternate tour: LA7

For more information

Los Angeles County Lifeguards, Southern Section (310) 372-2166
Marina del Rey Visitors' Center (310) 305-9545

TOUR LA4 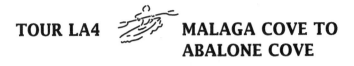 MALAGA COVE TO ABALONE COVE

Tour Details

Skill level:	Advanced
Trip length/type:	8.3 miles; one-way; open-ocean; two to three hours
Chart/map:	NOAA Chart #18744, 18746; USGS *Redondo Beach* 7.5 min series

Summary

Warm, sunny coves, craggy headlands, and forests of giant kelp teeming with sea life await you on this scenic ocean tour around the Palos Verdes Peninsula.

How to get there

To reach the launch site, exit the San Diego Freeway (Interstate 405) at Hawthorne Boulevard and proceed south to Palos Verdes Drive North. Go right to Palos Verdes Drive West. Go left to the first stop sign, Via Corta. Go right on Via Corta to Via Arroyo. Go right and park at the parking lot at the end of the road. There are no facilities and no fee.

To reach the landing site, exit the San Diego Freeway (Interstate 405) at Hawthorne Boulevard and proceed south to Palos Verdes Drive South. Go left to Abalone Cove and Shoreline Park, 5970 Palos Verdes Drive South. Parking, restrooms, telephones, seasonal lifeguard services, and picnic facilities are available. Fee.

Camping

There are no public campsites in the vicinity. For information about the nearest state park campground, call ParkNet 1-800-444-7275.

Hazards

Conditions are generally most hazardous north of Point Vicente. Between Point Vicente and Abalone Cove are several sheltered landing spots, but access to the beach from the bluff top is limited to steep, narrow trails. Avoid breaking and surging water when paddling around headlands. Localized thick kelp beds can make paddling difficult. Get an early start to be around Point Vicente before the afternoon winds pick up. Strong Santa Ana winds can occur any time of the year. Always be prepared for the possibility of fog.

Public access

The Palos Verdes Estates Shoreline Preserve, established in 1969, extends along the bluff top to the south of Malaga Cove. The preserve consists of 130 acres of undeveloped bluff-top park lands and submerged offshore lands. Several public footpaths lead from the bluff top to the rocky shoreline, but most of the trails are steep and narrow. Beach access is also available at Bluff Cove, Lunada Bay, and Point Vicente. Carrying a kayak to the water would be difficult at any of the above locations.

Kayak surfing

Good waves for kayak surfing can be found at Malaga Cove, Bluff Cove, and Lunada Bay.

Launching

A well-maintained, paved pathway leads from the parking lot at Malaga Cove to the beach. The beach is rocky and the waves can be strong, but usually break close to shore. A surf launch may be necessary. Launching is not recommended during periods of strong west or northwest swells. An alternate launch site is Redondo Beach King Harbor, approximately two and one-half miles north.

Tour description

From Malaga Cove, head southwest following the rocky shoreline. A gentle offshore breeze scented with sweet coastal sage whispers across the still, blue water. To the north is the Santa Monica Bay and the Santa Monica Mountains which stretch from Point Mugu to Elysian Park in Los Angeles. To the south, 20 miles off the coast, lies Santa Catalina Island.

The water visibility is usually good, and the bottom can be clearly seen at depths of up to 30 feet. Invertebrates such as scallops, sea hares, lobsters, rock crabs, and octopuses inhabit the rocky bottom. The beds of giant kelp provide the perfect habitat for garibaldi, sheephead, kelp bass, and rock fish. At the south end of Malaga Cove is a popular surf spot known as Haggarty's. The left-breaking waves are good for kayak surfing.

Approximately one mile southwest of Malaga Cove is Bluff Cove. Flat Rock and Bit Rock, two partly submerged rocks, lie about 100 yards offshore at the north end of the cove. Pass to seaward of the these rocks if there is a swell. Landing is possible at Bluff Cove during calm conditions. A dirt pathway leads from the bluff top to the beach. Bluff Cove is well known for its long, rolling waves, great for kayak surfing. At the south end of Bluff Cove is Indicator Point, another well-known surfing spot with left-breaking waves.

To the south of Bluff Cove is Palos Verdes Point (also known as Rocky Point), which is the most prominent headland between Malaga Cove and

Point Vicente. Palos Verdes Point has a long history of shipwrecks, the most recent in 1961 when the Greek Liberty Ship, *Dominator,* ran aground. The rusting remains can still be seen on the rocks at Palos Verdes Point.

At Palos Verdes Point the coastline turns southeast. Lunada Bay, just south of the point, is a wide, relatively shallow bay with thick kelp beds, supporting a variety of marine life. Harbor seals, pelicans, and cormorants can frequently be seen. The beach is rocky but landing is possible during calm conditions. Access is available to the bluff top via a steep, narrow trail. Good waves for kayak surfing can be found on the south side of the bay. Between Lunada Bay and Point Vicente are several smaller coves, and landing is possible during calm conditions, but access to the bluff top is limited.

About two and one-half miles southeast of Palos Verdes Point is Point Vicente. The point is an abrupt headland that marks a distinct bend in the coastline. Exposed in the face of the cliff are unique and colorful rock formations resulting from intense pressures and temperatures within the earth's crust. Frozen in time, these rocks now offer a unique picture of the geologic past.

To alert mariners of its ominous presence, a lighthouse was built on Point Vicente in 1926. Even with its warning beacon, the rocky headland is the graveyard for numerous shipwrecks. Submerged and partly submerged rocks which extend 250 yards offshore should always be given plenty of room when

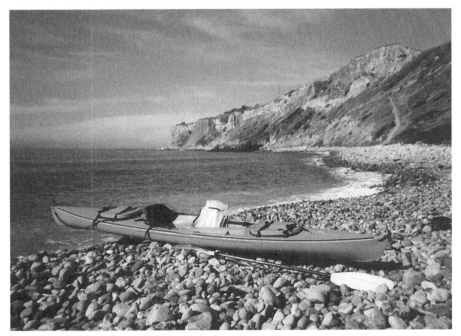

Landing site at Fisherman's Access, in the lee of Point Vicente

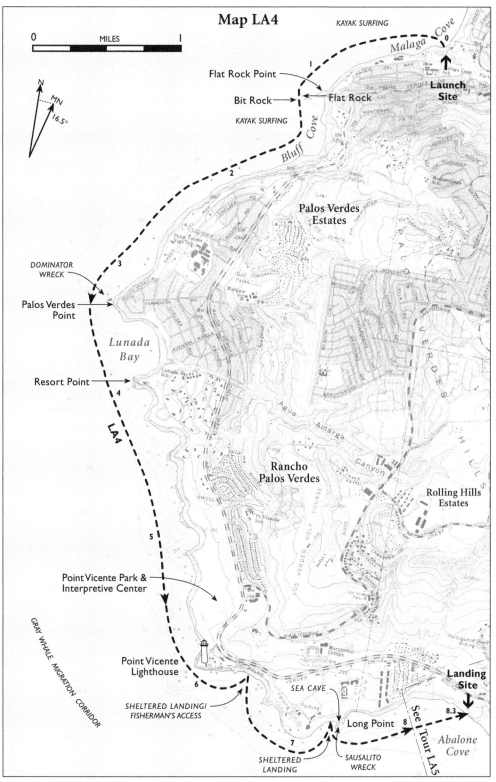

Map LA4

0   MILES   1

KAYAK SURFING

N
MN
16.5°

Flat Rock Point

Bit Rock   Flat Rock

KAYAK SURFING

Malaga Cove

Launch Site

Bluff Cove

1

2

Palos Verdes Estates

DOMINATOR WRECK

3

Palos Verdes Point

Lunada Bay

Resort Point

4

LA4

5

Rancho Palos Verdes

Agua Amarga Canyon

Rolling Hills Estates

Point Vicente Park & Interpretive Center

GRAY WHALE MIGRATION CORRIDOR

Point Vicente Lighthouse

6

Landing Site

SHELTERED LANDING/ FISHERMAN'S ACCESS

SEA CAVE

7   Long Point   8   8.3

See Tour LA5

Abalone Cove

SHELTERED LANDING

SAUSALITO WRECK

Tour LA4: Malaga Cove to Abalone Cove

rounding the point. The lighthouse, one of the most scenic on the California coast, is open to the public on a limited basis for guided tours. Point Vicente is a popular location for viewing California gray whales.

To the east of Point Vicente the wind and waves are usually much calmer. Landing is often possible at the Fisherman's Access, in the cove immediately east of the point. There is bluff-top parking and a steep dirt trail leading to the rocky beach.

The next major headland before you reach Abalone Cove is Long Point. The remains of the ship *Sausalito*, which went aground on the point are strewn across the beach. Parts of the wreck can also be seen in a large sea cave on the east side of the point.

Marineland of the Pacific, which at one time was the largest oceanarium in the world, was located on Long Point. The giant salt-water tank contained more than one million gallons of water and offered a variety of marine shows and attractions. Marineland closed in 1984 and the facility was demolished one year later. Abalone Cove is about one mile east of Long Point. The cove is relatively shallow and well-protected from the prevailing westerly winds and waves.

Landing

Land on the sandy beach in front of the lifeguard tower at Abalone Cove. The cove is sheltered from northwest winds and waves and conditions are usually favorable for landing. A surf landing may be necessary during a strong northwest or south swell. A steep dirt path leads from the beach to the parking area at the top of the bluff.

What to do afterward

The Point Vicente Park and Interpretive Center is about two miles west of Abalone Cove on Palos Verdes Drive South. The interpretive center, open daily, features a variety of geologic and marine displays. Artifacts excavated from a Gabrielino Indian village at Malaga Cove are also on display.

Alternate tour: LA7

For more information

Los Angeles County Lifeguards, Southern Section (310) 372-2166 (ask for Abalone Cove)

TOUR LA5 ABALONE COVE TO ROYAL PALMS STATE BEACH

Tour Details

Skill level:	Intermediate
Trip length/type:	4.5 miles; one-way; open-ocean; two to three hours
Chart/map:	NOAA Chart #18746; USGS *Redondo Beach* and *San Pedro* 7.5 min series

Summary

Sea caves, deserted beaches, and some of the best tide pools on the California coast make this an adventure you won't want to miss.

How to get there

To reach the launch site, exit the San Diego Freeway (Interstate 405) at Hawthorne Boulevard and proceed south to Palos Verdes Drive South. Go left to Abalone Cove and Shoreline Park, 5970 Palos Verdes Drive South. Parking, restrooms, telephones, seasonal lifeguard services, and picnic facilities are available. Fee.

To reach the landing site, exit the San Diego Freeway (Interstate 405) at Western Avenue and proceed south to the intersection of Western Avenue and Paseo del Mar in San Pedro. Follow the signs to Royal Palms State Beach. Parking, telephones, restrooms, and year-round lifeguard services are available. Fee.

Camping

There are no public campsites along the Palos Verdes shoreline. For information about the nearest state park campground, call ParkNet 1-800-444-7275.

Hazards

This section of coastline is somewhat protected from the westerly and northwesterly winds and waves by Point Vicente. Avoid breaking and surging water when passing around Portuguese and Inspiration points. There are several sheltered landing spots, but access to the beach from the bluff top is limited to steep, narrow trails. Localized, thick kelp beds can make paddling difficult. Strong Santa Ana winds can occur any time of the year. Always be prepared for the possibility of fog.

Public access

Most of the land between Abalone Cove Shoreline Park and Royal Palms State Beach is privately owned and public access is limited.

Kayak surfing

Good waves for kayak surfing can be found at Royal Palms State Beach.

Launching

Launch from the sand beach in front of the lifeguard tower at Abalone Cove. A steep dirt path leads from the parking area on the bluff top to the beach. The cove is sheltered from the northwest winds and waves and conditions are usually favorable for launching. A surf launch may be necessary during a strong northwest swell or south swell.

Tour description

Portuguese Point is located at the southeast end of Abalone Cove. As you paddle toward the point, notice the step-like appearance of the bluff and the reef extending offshore. This is a perfect example of a marine terrace in the process of being formed. Portuguese Point, which long ago was eroded level by wave action, has been uplifted to its present position as a marine terrace. The flat reef that extends off the end of the point is currently being eroded but will some day probably be uplifted to form a new terrace. Millions of years ago the Palos Verdes Peninsula was an island, uplifted from the sea floor. Sedimentation in the Los Angeles Basin caused the island to be connected to the mainland. As the peninsula was uplifted, a series of 13 marine terraces

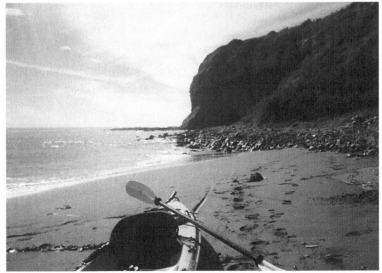

Smuggler's Cove served as a drop-off point for illegal spirits during Prohibition

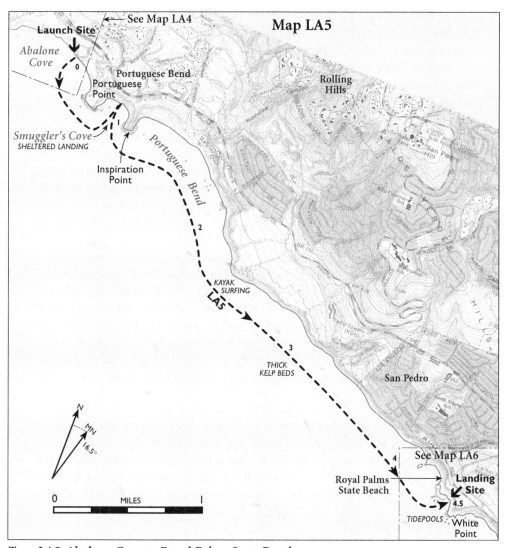

Tour LA5: Abalone Cove to Royal Palms State Beach

were cut by the waves. The process is ongoing, and today these step-like terraces can be clearly seen when viewing the profile of the Palos Verdes
Peninsula from a distance.

Portuguese Point and its sister Inspiration Point, located about one-quarter
mile to the east, both have beautiful tide pools to explore. The shallow pools
are filled with a variety of marine organisms including mussels, snails, hermit
crabs, limpets, barnacles, sea urchins, sea stars, sea anenomes, crabs, and octopuses. Portuguese Point has one sea cave and Inspiration Point has two. The
cave on Portuguese Point passes through the end of the point. If you plan on

exploring the sea caves, wear a helmet and a PFD and carry a waterproof flashlight. Always wait for a lull in the waves before entering a cave.

Separating Portuguese Point from Inspiration Point is Smuggler's Cove, also known a Sacred's Cove. Smuggler's Cove became well known during Prohibition, when it served as a drop-off point for illegal spirits. Today, the cove is a favorite spot for beachgoers. Protected by the prominent points on either side, the water is usually calm and suitable for landing.

To the southeast of Inspiration Point is Portuguese Bend, named for Portuguese whalers who operated a whaling station in the area during the mid 1800s. Grading operations for a highway built in 1956 triggered a large landslide in the area that continues to move at a rate of several inches per year and currently envelopes about 270 acres. Many exclusive homes have been damaged or lost as a result of the slide. Evidence of the slide is visible on the steep slopes above Portuguese Bend.

.To the east of the slide area is the Portuguese Bend Club, a private beach club with numerous facilities. Between the Portuguese Bend Club and Royal Palms are long, secluded, sand-and-cobble beaches. The bluffs are high and steep; access is limited to a few poorly maintained dirt trails. Most of the bluff top area is undeveloped and privately owned. Offshore, the kelp beds are very thick, and paddling can be difficult. The water is usually a murky blue-brown due to siltation from the Portuguese Bend slide. Good waves for kayak surfing can be found on some of the more prominent headlands.

Landing

Land on the small gravel-and-rock beach beyond the east end of the parking lot between Royal Palms State Beach and White Point. The waves are usually small and somewhat protected by the rocky reefs on either side of the beach. A surf landing may be necessary. If conditions are unfavorable, the next suitable landing site is Cabrillo Beach, about two and one-half miles southeast.

What to do afterward

The tide pools White Point are some of the most beautiful on the Palos Verdes Peninsula. Intensely folded rocks have formed a unique variety of tide pools capable of supporting a colorful assortment of tide-pool life including limpets, barnacles, urchins, sea stars, anenomes, hermit crabs and mussels. Offshore, an underwater marked nature trail has been developed for scuba divers.

Alternate tour: LA7

For more information

Los Angeles County Lifeguards, Southern Section (310) 372-2166
(ask for Abalone Cove or Royal Palms State Beach)

TOUR LA6   ROYAL PALMS STATE BEACH TO CABRILLO BEACH

Tour Details

Skill level:	Beginner
Trip length/type:	2.7 miles; one way; open-ocean; one to two hours
Chart/map:	NOAA Chart #18746; USGS *San Pedro* 7.5 min series

Summary

Spectacular views of the scenic Palos Verdes Peninsula and Catalina Island, thick kelp beds teeming with sea life, colorful tide pools, and the historic Point Fermin Lighthouse are all included in this kayaking adventure.

How to get there

To reach the launch site, exit the San Diego Freeway (Interstate 405) at Western Avenue and proceed south to the intersection of Western Avenue and Paseo del Mar in San Pedro. Follow the signs to Royal Palms State Beach. Parking, telephones, restrooms, picnic facilities, and year-round lifeguard services are available. Fee.

To reach the landing site exit the Harbor Freeway (Interstate 110) at Gaffey Street and proceed south to 22nd Street. Go left to Pacific Street. Go right to

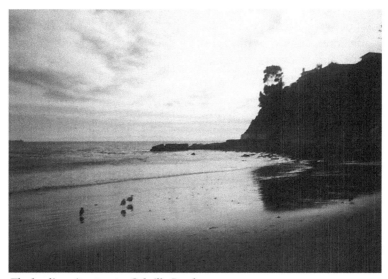

The landing site at outer Cabrillo Beach

36th Street (Stephen M. White Drive). Go left and park in the parking lot for the Cabrillo Marine Museum. Telephones, restrooms, picnic facilities, and year-round lifeguard services are provided. Fee.

Camping

There are no public campsites along the Palos Verdes shoreline. For information about the nearest state park campground, call ParkNet 1-800-444-7275.

Hazards

Avoid breaking and surging water when passing around Point Fermin and White Point. Strong winds and choppy, unsettled seas are common on the west side of Point Fermin during the afternoon. Much of the shoreline is rocky, with a wide, shallow reef extending offshore. Thick kelp beds can make paddling difficult. Strong Santa Ana winds can occur any time of the year. Always be prepared for the possibility of fog.

Public access

Public beach access is available at Wilder Annex, the western portion of Point Fermin Park, at the corner of Meyler Street and Paseo del Mar.

Kayak surfing

Good waves for kayak surfing can be found at Royal Palms State Beach, at Point Fermin, and at Cabrillo Beach.

Launching

Launch from the small gravel-and-rock beach beyond the east end of the parking lot between Royal Palms State Beach and White Point. The waves are usually small and somewhat protected by the rocky reefs on either side of the beach. A surf launch may be necessary.

Tour description

Royal Palms State Beach has an interesting history. In 1915 the Royal Palms Hotel was constructed on the beach. It was later destroyed by storms and an earthquake. The remains of the foundation and the palm trees for which the hotel was named can still be seen. At the south end of the beach is White Point. White Point Hot Springs and Spa, a Japanese-style resort hotel and bathhouse, was built in the early 1900s. The complex consisted of a natural sulfur hot spring, hotel, restaurant, and salt-water pool. The hot springs were fed by geothermal vents just offshore. The remains of the salt-water pool can be seen at low tide in the tide pools off White Point.

From the launch site paddle southeast around White Point. Watch for shallow submerged rocks off the end of the point. The beach east of White Point

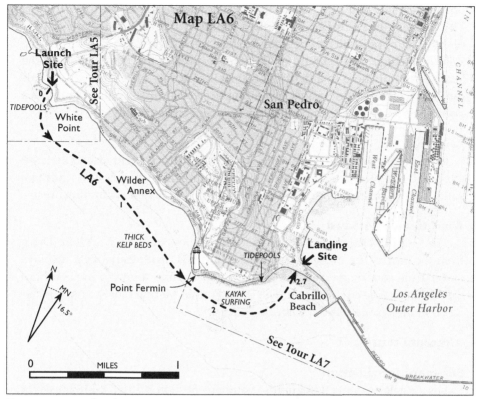

Tour LA6: Royal Palms State Beach to Cabrillo Beach

is narrow and rocky with a wide, shallow reef extending offshore; landing is not recommended. The bluff is high and steep, and the marine terrace is relatively narrow and developed with homes. Catalina Island, about 20 miles south, is visible on a clear day.

Point Fermin, at the east end of the Palos Verdes Peninsula, is about one and one-half miles southeast of White Point. The point is a bold headland exhibiting a distinct, horizontally bedded rock structure. Point Fermin was named in 1791 for Father Fermin Francisco de Lasuen, who established 9 of the 21 California missions. Standing high atop the bluff is the Point Fermin Lighthouse, built in 1874 on land purchased for $35.00 from Juan Sepulveda, one of the original Spanish Grant landowners in the Los Angeles area. The lighthouse was constructed from materials shipped by sailing vessels around Cape Horn. The original lighthouse operated until 1928, when an automated light was installed.

During the afternoon, strong winds can be encountered on the west side of Point Fermin. Fortunately, the prevailing westerly wind will be coming from behind you, which should make padding easier. To avoid the thick kelp beds on the west side of the point, you may want to paddle a little further offshore. The east side of Point Fermin is often sheltered from the wind and waves, offering an opportunity to explore the tide pools. The Point Fermin Marine Wildlife Refuge was established in 1969 to protect the marine life on the beaches and offshore to a depth of 600 feet. A variety of plants and animals can be seen in the tide pools, including acorn barnacles, hermit crabs, sea anenomes, sea urchins, limpets, sargasso weed, and surf grass.

Landing

Land on the west end of Cabrillo Beach near the point. The waves are usually small and break close to shore. A surf landing may be necessary during a south swell or a strong northwest swell. Avoid designated swimming areas.

What to do afterward

The Cabrillo Marine Aquarium is located across Stephen M. White Drive from the beach. The museum, established in 1934, features nautical displays and marine aquariums containing plants and animals found in the Southern California marine environment. The Point Fermin Marine Life Refuge is located on Point Fermin west of Cabrillo Beach.

Alternate tour: LA7

For more information

Los Angeles County Lifeguards, Southern Section (310) 372-2166 (ask for Royal Palms State Beach or Cabrillo Beach)

TOUR LA7 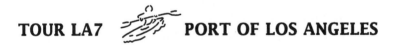 PORT OF LOS ANGELES

Tour Details	
Skill level:	Intermediate
Trip length/type:	6.5 miles; round-trip; harbor; three to four hours
Chart/map:	NOAA Chart #18746, 18749; USGS *San Pedro* 7.5 min series

Summary

Experience the sights and sounds of the Port of Los Angeles, the world's largest man-made harbor, on this action-packed adventure tour.

How to get there

To reach the launch site, exit the Harbor Freeway (Interstate 110) at Gaffey Street and proceed south to 22nd Street. Go left to Pacific Street. Go right to

36th Street (Stephen M. White Drive). Go left and park in the parking lot for the Cabrillo Marine Aquarium. Telephones, restrooms, picnic facilities, and year-round lifeguard services are available. Fee.

Camping

There are no public campsites in the vicinity. For information about the nearest state park campground, call ParkNet 1-800-444-7275.

Hazards

This tour is located within the Port of Los Angeles. Boat traffic can be congested; always follow the rules of the road. Be aware of fishing lines when paddling near docks or jetties. Gusty winds and choppy conditions are likely to be encountered in the outer harbor during the afternoon. Strong Santa Ana winds can occur any time of the year. Always be prepared for the possibility of fog.

Public access

The Port of Los Angeles is a "working" commercial harbor, and public access to docks or piers is restricted.

Kayak surfing

Good waves for kayak surfing can be found outside the breakwater at Cabrillo Beach.

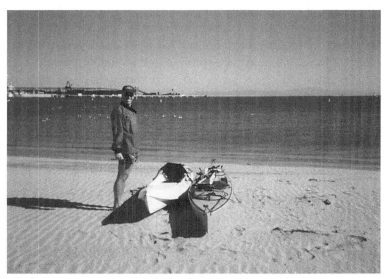

The launch site at inner Cabrillo Beach

Launching

Launch adjacent to the lifeguard station on the beach inside the breakwater at Cabrillo Beach. Conditions are calm and a surf landing will not be necessary. Stay clear of designated swimming areas.

Tour description

From Cabrillo Beach paddle east, about one-half mile across the West Channel, to the Union Bulk Terminal. The West Channel is often busy with boat traffic, so be observant and follow the rules of the road when crossing. The Union Bulk Terminal was constructed in 1960 to accommodate the large supertankers which were previously unable to enter the harbor. The facility has a loading capacity of 35,000 barrels of oil per hour. In December 1976, the 70,000-ton tanker *Sansinena* exploded and burned while unloading fuel at the dock. Nine persons were killed in the explosion, which I could hear from my house over 20 miles away.

From the south end of the Union Bulk Terminal head northeast toward the entrance to the Main Channel. On the left is a large iron-ore bulk-loading terminal. Mountains of stockpiled iron ore are loaded by conveyor belts into the holds of waiting ships.

At the entrance to the Main Channel is a large white building with *World Port Los Angeles* written across the side. The Port of Los Angeles Pilot Facility is located atop the building. Port pilots, stationed around the clock at the facility, are ferried to incoming and outgoing vessels to provide pilot services within the harbor. From the pilot facility, cross the Main Channel to Reservation Point, the southwest corner of Terminal Island. The large, white Coast Guard vessels moored at Reservation Point are used for rescuing stranded vessels at sea and apprehending drug traffickers. Adjacent to the Coast Guard base are several "floating dry docks" used to raise large ships out of the water for maintenance. The dock is first submerged by filling large ballast tanks with sea water. After a ship is maneuvered into the dock, the ballast tanks are pumped dry, raising the ship completely out of the water. Workers can then work on parts of the ship below the waterline. Continue along the east side of the channel past the tank farm and the container terminals. At the Vincent Thomas Bridge cross to the west side of the channel and head back toward the channel entrance.

The Vincent Thomas Bridge, connecting San Pedro with Terminal Island, was dedicated in 1963. It replaced the *Islander*, a ferry which had been in service since 1941. The bridge span rises 185 feet above the Main Channel and is over a mile long. Moored beneath the west end of the bridge is the *Lane Victory*, a World War II Victory Ship which has been refurbished and is open to the public. During World War II, hundreds of Victory Ships were used to transport troops and supplies overseas. Adjacent to the *Lane Victory* is the

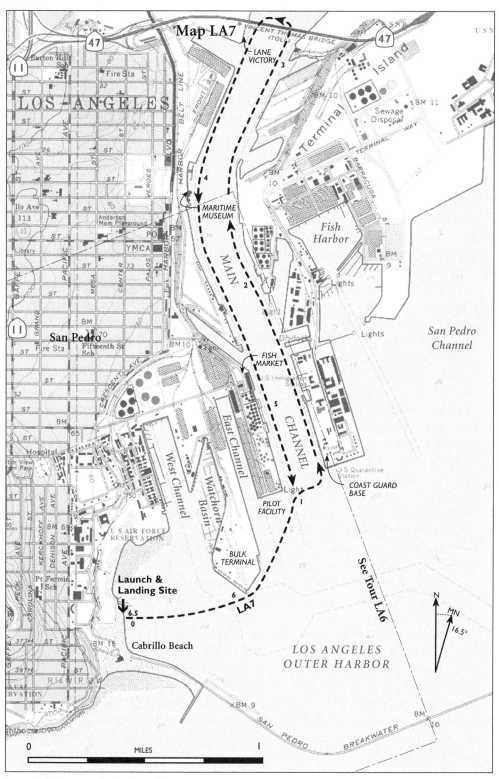

Tour LA7: Port of Los Angeles

Catalina Terminal, the point of departure for ferry services to Santa Catalina Island. Across a narrow channel from the Catalina Terminal is the World Cruise Center, home port for the "Love Boats." Paddling next to these floating cities can be a very humbling experience.

Next stop is the Port of Los Angeles Fire Station Number 1. Housed within the open-ended dome structure is the fire-fighting vessel, the *Bethel F. Gifford*. Crews are constantly on alert, ready to respond to a fire on a ship or at a port facility. South of the fire station is the Wrigley Tug Company. The small but powerful tugboats are used to maneuver large ships within the confines of the harbor. Stay clear of any vessel being assisted by a tug. Housed in the historic Municipal Ferry Building is the Los Angeles Maritime Museum. The museum contains ship models, nautical artifacts and a collection of photographs depicting the history of the Port of Los Angeles. Unfortunately there is not a guest dock for landing at the museum.

The area surrounding the Port of Los Angeles was originally settled by Shoshone-speaking native people, called Gabrielinos, who migrated westward from the Rocky Mountain area. They settled in villages throughout the San Pedro area and the Palos Verdes Peninsula. In 1542 the Portuguese explorer Juan Cabrillo sailed into San Pedro Bay aboard his flagship, the *San Salvador*. He named the bay Bahia de los Fumos, the "Bay of Smokes" perhaps due to fires set by the Gabrielinos to send signals. In 1602 the Spanish explorer Sebastian Vizcaino named the bay San Pedro. After the founding of the San Gabriel Mission in 1771, the Gabrielino people were gathered together and forced to work as laborers and to assist in ship loading.

In the early days, San Pedro Bay was unprotected and subject to southwest gales. Ships had to be anchored about a mile offshore for protection, and supplies were brought ashore by small boats which were landed precariously on the beach. The inner bay consisted of shallow lagoons and salt marshes. Richard Henry Dana in his book "Two Years Before the Mast" describes the early San Pedro as "the hell of California, and seemed designed in every way for the wear and tear of sailors." Since the 1870s, harbor improvements such as dredging, filling, and constructing breakwaters, have transformed the tidal flats and marshlands of San Pedro Bay into the largest artificial harbor in the world.

From the Maritime Museum, proceed south along Main Channel to Ports O' Call, a waterfront tourist village. The village is host to a variety of shops and several restaurants. Restrooms and telephones are available. South of Ports O' Call are the fisherman's dock and the San Pedro Fish Market. During unloading and processing of the day's catch, swarms of birds and an occasional hungry sea lion frantically compete for a handout. Continue south past the pilot facility and return to Cabrillo Beach. Strong headwinds may be encountered during the afternoon when crossing the West Channel from the super-tanker facility to Cabrillo Beach. If necessary, paddle north and cross the channel near the Cabrillo Marina.

Landing site and Landing

Land at Cabrillo Beach where you launched. Stay clear of designated swimming areas.

What to do afterward

The Cabrillo Marine Aquarium is across across the parking lot from the launch site. The museum, established in 1934, features nautical displays and marine aquariums containing plants and animals found in the Southern California marine environment. The Point Fermin Marine Life Refuge is located at Point Fermin, west of Cabrillo Beach.

Alternate tour: Tour LA8

For more information

Los Angeles County Lifeguards, Southern Section (310) 372-2166
Cabrillo Marine Aquarium (310) 548-7562

TOUR LA8 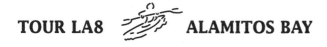 ALAMITOS BAY

Tour Details	
Skill level:	Beginner
Trip length/type:	5.5 miles; round-trip; bay; two to three hours
Chart/map:	NOAA Chart #18749; USGS *Long Beach, Los Alamitos* and *Seal Beach* 7.5 min series

Summary

Imagine yourself in Italy as you navigate through the narrow canals of Naples Island.

How to get there

To reach the launch site, exit the Long Beach Freeway (Interstate 710) at Ocean Boulevard and proceed east to Naples Landing, at 5437 East Ocean Boulevard on the Los Alamitos Peninsula. Park on the north side of Ocean Boulevard next to the City of Long Beach Sailing Center. Restrooms, picnic facilities, seasonal lifeguard services, a snack bar, kayak rentals, and telephones are available. No fee.

Camping

No camping facilities are available in the vicinity of Alamitos Bay. For information about the nearest state park campground, call ParkNet 1-800-444-7275.

Hazards

This tour is located entirely within Alamitos Bay. Boat traffic can be congested; always follow the rules of the road. Strong afternoon winds can make paddling difficult. Be aware of possible sharp underwater objects when exploring the shallow waters of the marshland area. Strong Santa Ana winds can occur at any time of the year. Always be prepared for the possibility of fog. If possible plan your trip route to have a following tidal current.

Public access

Most of the beaches surrounding Alamitos Bay are public but most of the docks and slips are privately owned. Several launch ramps are available for public use.

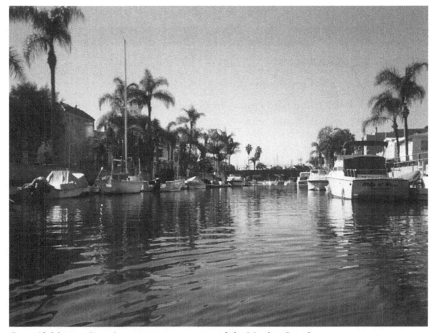

Beautiful homes line the narrow waterways of the Naples Canal

Kayak surfing

There are no waves for kayak surfing within Alamitos Bay. The closest beach for kayak surfing is Seal Beach, south of the Alamitos Bay entrance channel.

Launching

Launch from the boat ramp at Naples Landing. The sand beach is level and there are no waves.

Tour description

From Naples Landing head north along Alamitos Bay Beach, a narrow, sand, swimming beach. At approximately one-half mile, pass beneath the Second Street bridge. The pilings beneath the bridge have been painted by the local college rowing teams with slogans announcing the various championships won over the years. Just beyond the Second Street bridge is the Long Beach Marine Stadium, constructed during the 1920s and used for the rowing races held during the 1932 Olympic Games in Los Angeles. The stadium is a two-mile-long, rectangular body of water used today for water skiing and boat racing. Carefully cross the marine stadium, watching for passing boats, and continue northeast into the Los Cerritos Channel. On the left is a large boat marina and residential development and on the right are private boat docks and restaurants.

At about one-quarter mile northwest of the marine stadium is the Highway 1 bridge. After you pass beneath the bridge, the Cerritos Bahia Marina will be on the left and the Los Cerritos Wetlands on the right. A full-size metal sculpture of a man fishing from the shore marks the entrance to the wetlands. From the main channel proceed to the right into the wetlands area.

The Los Cerritos Wetlands, which extend from the Los Cerritos Channel to the San Gabriel River, are the only remaining natural habitat of the once-extensive Alamitos Bay marshlands. A variety of shore and land birds, including the endangered California least tern, can be observed nesting in the marsh grass. Considering their location, surrounded by busy highways, shopping malls, oil fields, and power plants, the wetlands are a surprisingly tranquil spot. Paddle through the narrow tidal channels, being careful not to disturb the wildlife. Imagine how it was when the Gabrielino Indians hunted and fished and thousands of migratory birds nested in the once-expansive marshlands.

Return to the Los Cerritos Channel and head southwest, back to the marine stadium. When you reach the stadium, turn left and continue clockwise around Naples Island. On the left are a group of condominiums and a public launch ramp and on the right is a sand beach. Pass beneath the Second Street bridge and enter the Long Beach Marina, home of several exclusive yacht

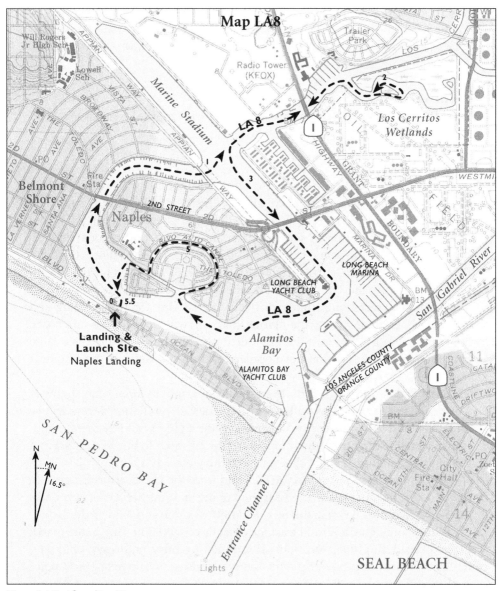

Tour LA8: Alamitos Bay

clubs and thousands of pleasure craft. On the left, just beyond the bridge, are the marina shipyard and a marine rescue facility. The large building on the right is the Long Beach Yacht Club. Across the channel is the Seal Beach Yacht Club.

At the Long Beach Yacht Club, the channel turns to the southwest; ahead is the entrance channel to Alamitos Bay. On the east side of the entrance channel is Seaport Village, a tourist attraction with shops and restaurants. On the west side of the entrance channel is the Alamitos Peninsula, a residential beach community with public walkways and a bike path. The Alamitos Bay Yacht Club is at the southeast tip of the peninsula.

Follow the shoreline of Naples Island until you reach the entrance to the Naples Canal. Turn right into the narrow canal and proceed counterclockwise around the loop, which winds through the interior of the island. Naples Island actually consists of three small islands that were constructed in the early 1900s. The islands were formed with pilings and retaining walls and were filled with material dredged from the marshland. Today, the island is developed, with beautiful homes crowded along the narrow waterways. It's easy to imagine yourself in Italy, as you pass beneath the low-arched bridges and watch the authentic gondolas slip silently past. Exit the canal and cross the channel to Naples Landing.

Landing
Land at the boat ramp at Naples Landing where you launched.

What to do afterward
The *Queen Mary* is about three miles west of Naples Landing at Pier J, off the Long Beach 710 Freeway. The former British luxury liner made more than 1000 transatlantic voyages before being moved to her present home in Long Beach. The *Queen Mary* is now a tourist attraction housing numerous shops and restaurants, and a hotel. At Christmas time, Naples has a wonderful light-ed boat parade. Get some lights for your kayak and plan on entering the parade.

Alternate tour: LA7

For more information
City of Long Beach, Department of Parks, Recreation and Marine
(562) 570-3100

Orange County Tours

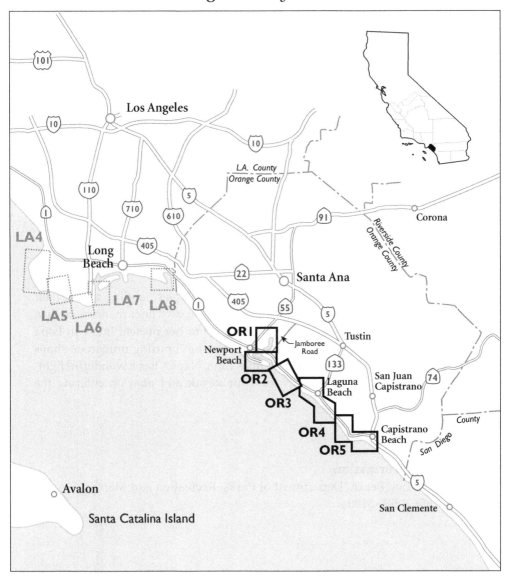

Tour	Skill Level	Length
OR1: Upper Newport Bay	Beginner	5.8 miles
OR2: Newport Harbor	Beginner	6.7 miles
OR3: Newport Harbor to Reef Point	Intermediate	4.5 miles
OR4: Reef Point to Aliso County Beach	Intermediate	6.5 miles
OR5: Aliso County Beach to Doheny State Beach	Advanced	6.8 miles

Chapter 8

Orange County

I had been to Newport Beach numerous times over the years but I had never experienced it like this. Our kayaks glided across the glassy evening water as we paddled past row after row of magnificent yachts—everything from square-rigged schooners to refurbished tugboats. Newport Harbor has about every kind of yacht imaginable.

My friend, who had grown up in Newport Beach, was the perfect guide. As we paddled along Lido Isle Reach toward the Turning Basin, he pointed out all the fancy restaurants; each with its own private landing dock to service anyone who preferred to go to dinner in a boat rather than a car. Up ahead on the right was the Wild Goose, *which at one time belonged to John Wayne, and was now an excursion boat catering to private parties.*

We paddled beneath the bridge to Lido Isle and headed east along the Balboa Peninsula passing the Newport Yacht Club and the famous Balboa Pavilion, a distinctive Victorian style building that was a dance hall during the 1940s and was restored in 1962. The harbor was alive with activity. Big boats and small boats moving in every direction. It was hard to imagine where they all could be going. A small skiff passed by with a couple of kids hanging over the side. They were feeding a huge male sea lion that was barking loudly every time they threw him a fish.

We crossed the channel and headed west along Balboa Island. The western sky was a deep crimson and the stars, one by one, appeared in the fading light. The buzz of activity so prevalent just a short while ago was replaced by a hushed silence.

The lights of the Pavilion reflected across the smooth surface of the bay. The Wild Goose *slowly passed and the sound of music and laughter drifted across the water. A couple leaning over the stern waved to us then vanished into the night.*

— Newport Harbor, March 22, 1997

TOUR OR1 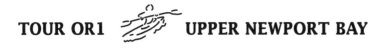 UPPER NEWPORT BAY

Tour Details

Skill level:	Beginner
Trip length/type:	5.8 miles; round-trip; bay; two to three hours
Chart/map:	NOAA Chart #18754; USGS *Newport Beach* 7.5 min series

Summary

Pastel colors of the setting sun reflected off the chalky cliffs of Dover Heights; silver moonlight dancing across the calm water; and the silhouette of sea birds against the glistening mud flats are just a part of the magic you will experience on a moonlight tour of the Upper Newport Bay Ecological Reserve.

How to get there

To reach the launch site exit the San Diego Freeway (Interstate 405) at Jamboree Road and proceed south about five miles to Backbay Drive (about one block north of Pacific Coast Highway/Highway 1. Turn right on Backbay Drive and enter the Newport Dunes Resort. Parking, restrooms, picnic facilities, telephones, kayak rentals and tours, and lifeguard services are available. Fee.

Camping

Tent and RV campsites are available at the Newport Dunes Resort. For reservations call (800) 288-0770.

Hazards

This tour is entirely within Upper Newport Bay. Boat traffic can be congested; follow the rules of the road at all times. Plan your trip so you will be paddling *with* the tidal current and so you can explore the estuary during an incoming, high tide. Getting stuck in the mud flats is not fun. Strong Santa Ana winds can occur at any time of the year. Always be prepared for the possibility of fog.

Public access

Public access on the west side of the bay is available at North Star Beach, adjacent to the Newport Aquatic Center, on North Star Lane off Polaris Drive.

Kayak surfing

There are no waves for kayak surfing within Upper Newport Bay.

Launching

Launch from the sand beach at the Newport Dunes Resort. The launch site is within the bay and there are no waves. Avoid designated swimming areas.

Tour description

Upper Newport Bay is a wide, flat, north/south-trending estuary bordered on the east and west by high vertical cliffs. The estuary is undeveloped except for Backbay Drive, a one-way road that follows the eastern shoreline of the bay. The bluff tops surrounding the bay are developed with residences. On the hills to the east, overlooking the bay, are the lofty high-rise buildings of Newport Fashion Island. Newport Harbor is to the south.

About one million years ago, when sea level was much lower than it is today, Upper Newport Bay was a deep canyon, carved out of the surrounding bedrock by the Santa Ana River. As sea level rose, sediment filled the canyon, creating the estuary we see today. Prior to the mid-1800s, Upper Newport Bay was connected directly to the Pacific Ocean. During flooding in 1861, the Santa Ana River deposited an offshore sand spit which formed the Balboa Peninsula, cutting the Upper Bay off from direct ocean influence. In 1917, as part of the development of Newport Harbor, the Santa Ana River was diverted from the bay to its present location about three miles to the west. Work continued on the harbor until 1936, when it was officially dedicated as a small boat harbor.

From the Newport Dunes paddle north, passing beneath the narrow pedestrian bridge. On the east bank, just past the bridge, are the Newport Dunes boat ramp and the University of California at Irvine rowing facility. The calm

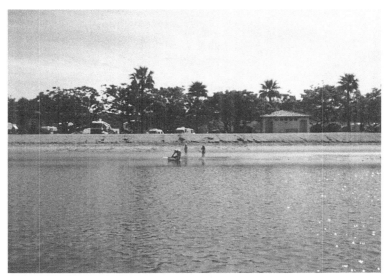

Launching at the Newport Dunes Resort

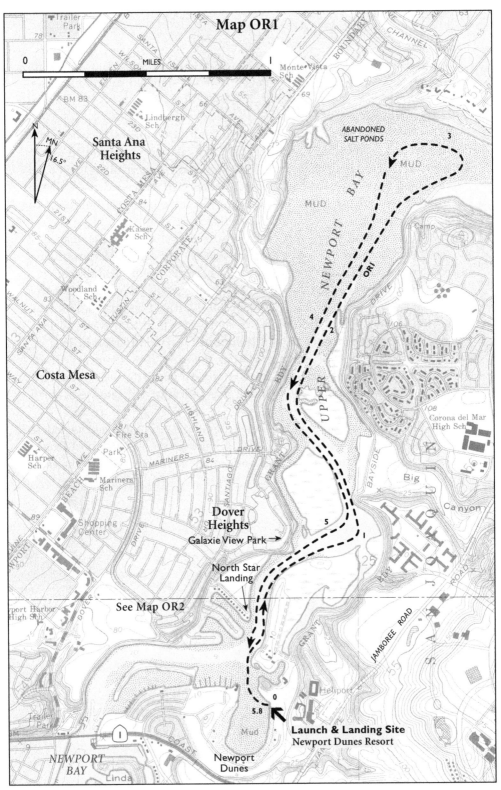

Tour OR1: Upper Newport Bay

waters of the bay are training areas for several rowing teams. Across the channel on the west bank are condominiums and boat docks. Just north of the condominiums are the Newport Beach Aquatic Center and North Star Beach. About one-half mile ahead are the distinctive white cliffs of Dover Heights.

North of Dover Heights, the channel turns in a broad S-curve. Bicyclists can be seen riding along Backbay Drive, which parallels the eastern shoreline. The water is usually smooth and the air still, but the peaceful setting is occasionally interrupted by noisy jets departing from nearby John Wayne International Airport.

Established as an ecological reserve in 1975, Upper Newport Bay contains 752 acres of tidal channels, mud flats, and salt marshes. It is one of the few remaining estuaries in Southern California and is the home of up to 30,000 birds, including six endangered species. The marshland is a unique environment where fresh water and salt water mix. Vegetation varies depending upon the extent of tidal exposure and the salinity of the water. The intertidal mud flats are vegetated with eel grass and sea weed while the salt marshes, which border the mud flats, are vegetated with cord grass, salt grass, and pickle weed. Although few bird species inhabit coastal wetlands year-round, many species inhabit the wetlands during their annual migrations. Coastal California is part of the Pacific Flyway, one of the four principal bird migration routes in North America. During the winter months, thousands of migratory birds including willets, plovers, sandpipers, and shovelers stop to rest and feed in the sheltered environment of the upper bay. The mud flats are also the perfect environment for a host of invertebrates such as clams, snails, and bay mussels. Deep-sea fish such as halibut, white croaker, and white seabass utilize the warm, shallow water as a spawning ground and nursery.

About two miles north of the launch site, the mud flats broaden and the channel turns east. Jamboree Road, which crosses the marshland east of the bay, can be seen ahead. This part of the bay was operated as an elaborate saltworks plant from 1934 until 1969, when the evaporation ponds were destroyed by flooding. Continue to follow the tidal channel but test the water depth frequently with your paddle to avoid getting stuck in the mud. When the water becomes about two feet deep, turn around and return to Newport Dunes Resort, following the same route.

Landing

Land at Newport Dunes Resort where you launched. Avoid designated swimming areas.

What to do afterward

Educational walks, kayak, and canoe tours of Upper Newport Bay are offered by the Upper Newport Bay Naturalists, an all-volunteer organization that is committed to restoring and protecting the fragile environment of the estuary.

Alternate tour: OR2

For more information
Newport Beach Harbor Patrol (714) 723-1002
Upper Newport Bay Naturalists (714) 640-6746

TOUR OR2 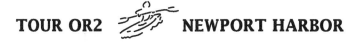 NEWPORT HARBOR

Tour Details	
Skill level:	Beginner
Trip length/type:	6.7 miles; round-trip; bay; three to four hours
Chart/map:	NOAA Chart #18754; USGS *Newport Beach* 7.5 min series

Summary
Square-rigged schooners, world-class racing yachts, spectacular bay-front mansions and fine waterfront restaurants are just a sample of the sights to be seen on this round-trip tour of Newport Harbor.

How to get there
To reach the launch site, exit the San Diego Freeway (Interstate 405) at the Newport Freeway (Highway 55) and proceed south to Newport Beach, where the Newport Freeway (Newport Boulevard) merges with Balboa Boulevard. Turn left on 18th Street and go one block to West Bay Avenue. Park in the metered street parking on West Bay Avenue. Restrooms and telephones are available. No fee, but bring plenty of quarters for the parking meter (one dollar per hour/six hours limit). Free parking is available on the adjoining streets if you are fortunate enough to find an open space. Annual parking permits, which are valid for this location, are available from the city of Newport Beach.

Camping
Tent and RV campsites are available at the Newport Dunes Resort. For reservations call (800) 288-0770.

Hazards
This tour is entirely within Newport Bay. Boat traffic can be congested; follow the rules of the road at all times. If possible plan your trip so you will be

paddling *with* the tidal current and afternoon wind. Strong Santa Ana winds can occur at any time of the year. Always be prepared for the possibility of fog.

Public access
Most of the shoreline in Newport Harbor is privately owned. Parking is limited.

Kayak surfing
Waves for kayak surfing can be found outside the harbor entrance, but avoid the "Wedge," a well-known body-surfing spot located on the west side of the harbor entrance.

Launching
Launch from the sand beach at West Bay Avenue. There are no waves.

Tour description
From the launch site proceed east, following the shoreline of the Balboa Peninsula. Stay between the beach and the private yachts anchored just off-shore. Across the channel is Lido Island.

The Balboa Peninsula is a three-mile-long sand spit separating Newport Harbor from the Pacific Ocean. The entrance to the harbor is at the southeast end of the peninsula. The shoreline is fully developed with residential and commercial structures. Most of the residences have private boat docks on the waterfront. There are several public beaches but parking is limited.

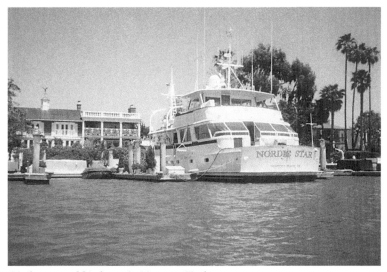

Big homes and big boats in Newport Harbor

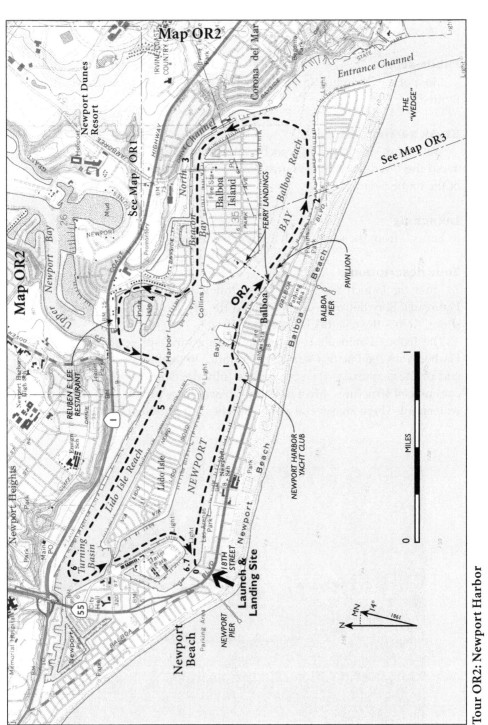

Tour OR2: Newport Harbor

About one mile east of the launch site is Newport Harbor Yacht Club. Just east of the yacht club is Bay Island, a tiny island developed with several homes. Pass beneath the pedestrian bridge separating Bay Island and the Balboa Peninsula. The island has no roads, and residents must park their cars in a parking lot on the peninsula and walk across the footbridge.

From Bay Island continue along the peninsula past the Ferry Landing to the Balboa Pavilion. The historic Victorian structure, which served as a dance hall throughout the 1940s, was restored in 1962 and now is a central tourist attraction for Newport Beach. At night the brightly lit Pavilion casts a sparkling reflection across the quiet waters of the bay.

Follow the shoreline of the Balboa Peninsula for another one-half mile, then cross the Main Channel and enter Balboa Island North Channel, which separates Balboa Island from the mainland. On the right as you enter the North Channel are the US Coast Guard facility, the Harbor Master offices, and two private yacht clubs. Follow the channel around the north side of Balboa Island to Harbor Island. Harbor Island has the reputation as being the most valuable real estate in the world. Beautiful mansions line the shore. On the east end of the island is a sprawling estate with beautifully landscaped grounds, waterfalls, and its very own lighthouse. Perhaps John Wayne, James Cagney, or Errol Flynn, long-time Newport Beach residents, lived there at one time.

Pass beneath the bridge separating Harbor Island and the mainland and follow the narrow channel around Linda Isle. When you reach the *Reuben E. Lee*, a floating riverboat which serves as a restaurant, turn left and head back to the Main Channel.

Turn right at the Main Channel and head west. The mainland is on the right and Lido Island is on the left. Yachts of all shapes and sizes are moored at the private docks along the shoreline. On the right is the Balboa Bay Club. Near the turning basin at the end of the channel are numerous fine restaurants and bars. Most have guest landing docks. On your right look for *Wild Goose,* which at one time belonged to John Wayne. *Wild Goose* is now an excursion boat catering to private parties.

From the turning basin at the west end of the Main Channel, pass beneath the bridge connecting Lido Island to the mainland and return to the landing site at West Bay Avenue.

Landing

Land on the sand beach at West Bay Avenue where you launched.

What to do afterward

The Newport Beach Pier, just a two blocks west of 19th Street, is the oldest pier in Southern California. The Newport Dory Fishing Fleet, founded in 1891, still launches every morning from the north side of the pier.

Alternate tour: OR1

For more information
Newport Beach Harbor Patrol (714) 723-1002

TOUR OR3 NEWPORT HARBOR TO REEF POINT (CRYSTAL COVE STATE PARK)

Tour Details

Skill level:	Intermediate
Trip length/type:	4.5 miles; one-way; open ocean; two to three hours
Chart/map:	NOAA Chart #18746; USGS *Newport Beach* and *Laguna Beach* 7.5 min series

Summary

Natural rock arches, undeveloped shoreline and long stretches of white sand beaches provide a sense of freedom and adventure on this tour of the Orange County coastline.

How to get there

To reach the launch site, exit the San Diego Freeway (Interstate 405) at Jamboree Road and proceed south about five and one-half miles to Bayside Drive (one block south of Pacific Coast Highway/Highway 1). Turn left and go to Bayside Drive County Beach, adjacent to the Orange County Sheriff Station and Harbor Patrol facility at 1901 Bayside Drive. Limited street parking, restrooms, showers, and picnic facilities, are available. No fee.

To reach the landing site, exit Pacific Coast Highway/Highway 1 south of Newport Beach at Reef Point Road in Crystal Cove State Park. Park at the south end of the parking lot. Restrooms, picnic facilities, and telephones are available. Fee.

Camping

Tent and RV campsites are available at Crystal Cove State Park. For camping reservations, call ParkNet (800) 444-7275.

Hazards

Give all headlands and shoals plenty of room during high seas. Boat traffic can be congested in the entrance channel to Newport Harbor; follow the rules of the road at all times. Strong Santa Ana winds can occur at any time of the year. Always be prepared for the possibility of fog.

Public access

Most of the shoreline between Newport Harbor and Crystal Cove State Park is public but the bluff is steep and access to the beach is difficult. Public parking and access to the beach within the park are available at Pelican Point, Los Trancos, and Reef Point.

Kayak surfing

Good waves for kayak surfing can be found at Reef Point.

Launching

Launch from the sandy beach at Bayside Drive County Beach. Kayaks must be transported a short distance from the street to the launch site. Although the launch site is within Newport Harbor, afternoon chop and boat wake can generate small waves. Launching of manual-powered boats only is allowed. Launch hours are restricted on weekends and during the summer.

Tour description

From Bayside Drive County Beach paddle south toward the Newport Harbor Entrance Channel. On the left is the old Irvine family boathouse. In

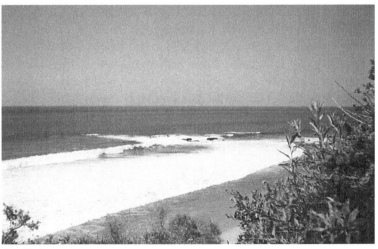

Reef Point

the early 1860s James Irvine, a Scottish immigrant, purchased Rancho San Joaquin from Jose Sepulveda. The vast land holdings, which were part of the original Mexican land grant, made Irvine the largest landowner in the area. The bright-blue building on the waterfront no longer serves as the Irvines' boathouse, but the Irvine Company still has vast land holdings and commercial interests in the Orange County area.

On the east side of the Entrance Channel is Rocky Point, a picturesque rock outcrop formerly known as Pirate's Cove. Conditions are usually calm enough for landing on the beach. The cove is noted for its clear water and good diving. Outside the west jetty is the "Wedge," a body-surfing spot famous for its treacherous, pounding waves.

From the harbor mouth head southeast. Abalone Point, about four miles southeast, is visible on a clear day. Just south of the entrance-channel jetty is Corona del Mar State Beach. The community of Corona del Mar is located on the bluff top above the beach. At the south end of Corona del Mar State Beach is Little Corona del Mar Beach, known for its rich tide pools. Folded and faulted rock formations provide the perfect habitat for an abundance of diverse organisms. A surf landing may be necessary if you choose to go ashore.

To the south of Little Corona del Mar is Crystal Cove State Park. The State of California purchased the land from the Irvine Company in 1979, and the Department of Parks and Recreation began managing the land in 1982. The park encompasses 2,971 acres of land with 3.5 miles of undeveloped shoreline extending from Coronal del Mar to Laguna Beach. Most of the shoreline is exposed to the westerly wind and waves; a surf landing is often necessary. The narrow, sandy beach is backed by a high sandstone bluff vegetated with coastal sage scrub. Offshore, a 1,140-acre underwater park has been created within the boundaries of the state park. The underwater park is fully protected under the Fish and Game Wildlife Refuge Act.

Just within the northern boundary of Crystal Cove State Park is Pelican Point, a scenic rocky headland. Powerful waves have eroded the intensely folded shale beds, creating numerous sea caves and natural rock arches. Watch for shallow rocks and breaking waves when approaching the point.

Southeast of Pelican Point is the Crystal Cove Historic District. Originally known as Tent City, the small coastal community was managed by Irvine Ranch employees. In the 1940s the tents were replaced by bungalows and cottages. The unique community has remained unchanged over the years and has served as a backdrop for numerous movies. The 46 cottages have recently been added to the National Register of Historic Places and are intended for public rental in the future.

The next headland is Reef Point. A partly submerged reef extends approximately two hundred yards offshore. Good waves for kayak surfing can be found on the northwest side of the reef. Tide pools can be explored during calm conditions. Stay to seaward of all breaking waves when passing the reef.

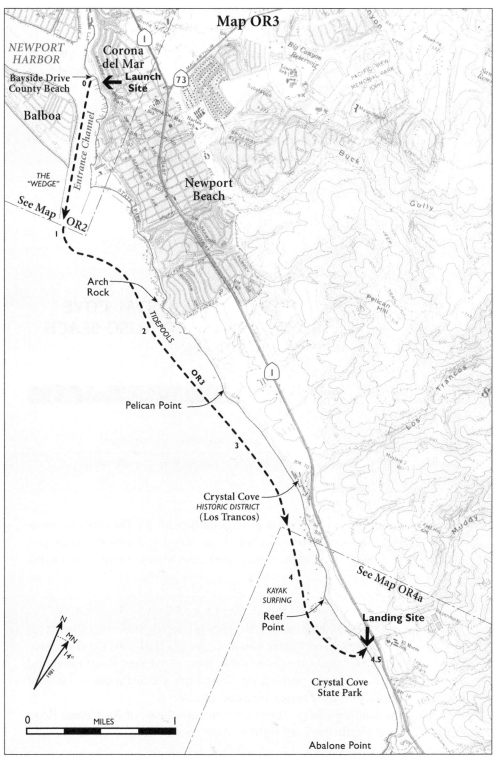

Trip OR3: Newport Harbor to Reef Point (Crystal Cove State Park)

Landing
Land on the sand beach south of Reef Point. A paved footpath leads from the beach to the south end of the parking lot at Reef Point. Be prepared for a surf landing. Watch for rocks in the surf zone.

What to do afterward
Crystal Cove State Park offers a variety of outdoor activities including hiking, biking, horseback riding, fishing, swimming, surfing, and diving.

Alternate tour: OR1 or OR2

For more information
Crystal Cove State Park, Ranger Headquarters (714) 494-3539

TOUR OR4 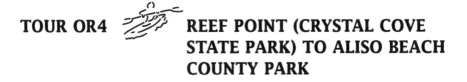 REEF POINT (CRYSTAL COVE STATE PARK) TO ALISO BEACH COUNTY PARK

Tour Details	
Skill level:	Intermediate
Trip length/type:	6.5 miles; one-way; open-ocean; three to four hours
Chart/map:	NOAA Chart #18746; USGS *Laguna Beach* 7.5 min series

Summary
Tired of fighting the traffic jams in Laguna Beach? Try the offshore route and you'll be surprised at what you have been missing. Along the route you will stop at secluded coves, explore tide pools, and visit a colony of sea lions.

How to get there
To reach the launch site, exit the the San Diego Freeway (Interstate 405) at Laguna Canyon Road (Highway 133) and go seven miles southwest to Laguna Beach. Turn right on Pacific Coast Highway/Highway 1 and go three miles northwest to Crystal Cove State Park. Turn left at Reef Point Road and park at the south end of the parking lot. Restrooms, picnic facilities, seasonal lifeguard services, and telephones are available. Fee

To reach the landing site go about six miles southeast of Reef Point Road on Pacific Coast Highway. Turn right at Aliso Beach County Park. Metered parking, restrooms, picnic facilities, lifeguard services, and telephones are available. No fee.

Camping

Tent and RV campsites are available at Crystal Cove State Park. For camping reservations, call ParkNet (800) 444-7275.

Hazards

This section of coastline has numerous rocky headlands and shallow offshore reefs, and rocks. Use caution when approaching and passing these potential hazards. Strong Santa Ana winds can occur at any time of the year. Always be prepared for the possibility of fog.

Public access

Northwest of Laguna Beach, public access to the beach is limited (except at Heisler Park). South of Main Beach the beach is accessible from most of the street ends, but parking is limited and the stairways to the beach are narrow and steep. Transportation of a kayak to the beach would be difficult.

Kayak surfing

Good waves for kayak surfing can be found at Heisler Park (Rock Pile Beach), Halfway Rock, and at Treasure Island Point.

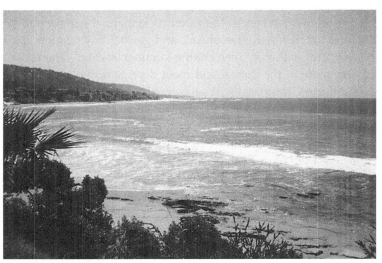

Looking south from the bluff at Heisler Park

Launching

Launch from the sand beach south of Reef Point. A paved footpath leads from the south end of the bluff-top parking lot at Reef Point to the beach. A surf launch is often necessary. Watch for rocks in the surf zone.

Tour description

From Reef Point head south, following the relatively straight shoreline. The sand beach is narrow and backed by a steep bluff vegetated with coastal sage, scrub plants, and chaparral. The hillsides to the northeast are mostly undeveloped. Before the arrival of the Spanish, the Gabrielino Indians inhabited the area, and the remnants of several villages have been found within Crystal Cove State Park.

About one mile southeast of Reef Point is Abalone Point, a prominent headland with a shallow reef extending offshore. Approach the point carefully and watch for submerged rocks. On the lee side of the point are several large sea caves, accessible only on very calm days.

Southeast of Abalone Point the shoreline is rugged with rocky headlands, shallow reefs, and offshore rocks. Nestled between closely spaced headlands are sheltered coves with narrow sand beaches. Irvine Cove and Emerald Bay are both private beaches inaccessible to the public. Huge mansions, resembling those of the French Riviera, stair-step up the steeply sloping hillsides.

South of Emerald Bay is Two Rock Point. Seal Rock, one of the two large offshore rocks, is inhabited by a colony of sea lions. Their loud barking can be heard nearly a mile away. Crescent Bay Point Park, overlooking Seal Rock, is a favorite spot for whale watching and wedding ceremonies.

The Laguna Beach Marine Wildlife Refuge extends from Two Rock Point to the northern end of Main Beach. The water is clear and the rocky bottom is the perfect habitat for rock fish, sheephead, and garibaldi. Common and bottlenose dolphins are frequently seen during summer and fall. The rocky shoreline supports some of the richest and most diverse tide-pool populations in Southern California. Intertidal species commonly seen include mussels, barnacles, anemones, chitons, hermit crabs, urchins, and sea stars. Within the refuge is the 30-acre Glenn E. Vedder Ecological Reserve. Collecting of tide-pool organisms is prohibited within the Laguna Beach Marine Wildlife Refuge.

Just northwest of Laguna Main Beach are several small coves with public access off Cliff Drive. Landing is possible during calm conditions. Heisler Park has restrooms, outdoor showers, and picnic facilities. Good waves for kayak surfing can be found at Rock Pile Beach just below the park. A paved trail leads from Heisler Park to Main Beach.

Southeast of Main Beach is a long, straight, sand beach. The bluff is high and developed with residences, condominiums, and hotels. Many of the beach-front properties are supported by sea walls, which have been painted

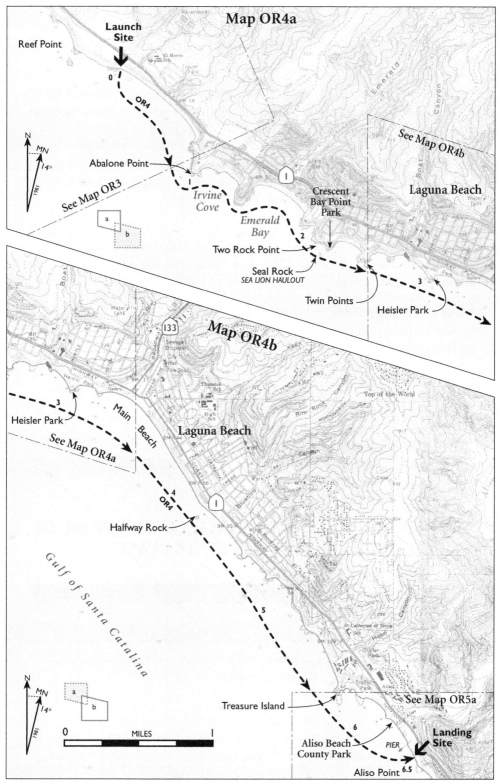

Trip OR4: Reef Point (Crystal Cove State Beach) to Aliso Beach County Park

with huge murals depicting the marine environment. Landing is possible and the beach is accessible from the bluff top but parking is limited. The stairways to the beach are steep and narrow, difficult for transporting a kayak.

Halfway Rock is a partly submerged rock lying about one hundred yards offshore. The waves break well offshore and can be good for kayak surfing. South of Halfway Rock the sandy beach is interrupted by occasional rocky reefs and small headlands. An exposed rock reef at Treasure Island shelters a small beach and cove. Good waves for kayak surfing break off the end of the reef. Landing in the cove is possible during calm conditions. The pier at Aliso Beach County Park can be seen from Treasure Island.

Landing

Land on the sand beach adjacent to the pier at Aliso Beach County Park. A surf landing may be necessary. This site has a very hazardous shorebreak when the waves a large.

What to do afterward

Laguna Beach is a popular beach community with numerous shops and art galleries featuring local artists.

Alternate tour: OR1 or OR2

For more information

Laguna Beach Lifeguards (714) 494-6571

Laguna Beach Weather (714) 494-6573

Crystal Cove State Park, Ranger Headquarters (714) 494-3539

TOUR OR5 ALISO BEACH COUNTY PARK TO DOHENY STATE BEACH

Tour Details	
Skill level:	Advanced
Trip length/type:	6.8 miles; one-way; open-ocean; three to four hours
Chart/map:	NOAA Chart #18746; USGS *Laguna Beach, San Juan Capistrano* and *Dana Point* 7.5 min series

Summary

In his well-known book *Two Years Before the Mast*, Richard Henry Dana, Jr. described Dana Point as the "only romantic spot on the coast." Although much has changed since Dana visited the point as a seaman on the brig *Pilgrim* in 1835, this trip still offers a taste of romance and excitement to anyone with an adventurous spirit.

How to get there

To reach the launch site, exit the San Diego Freeway (Interstate 405) at Laguna Canyon Road (Highway 133) and go seven miles southwest to Laguna Beach. Turn left on Pacific Coast Highway/Highway 1 and go about two and one-half miles southeast to Aliso Beach County Park. Turn right at Aliso Beach County Park. Metered parking, restrooms, picnic facilities, lifeguard services, and telephones are available. No fee.

To reach the landing site, exit the San Diego Freeway (Interstate 5) at Pacific Coast Highway/Highway 1 in Capistrano Beach. Go west to Dana Point Harbor Drive. Go left on Dana Point Harbor Drive to Park Lantern. Go left to Doheny State Beach. Park in the north, day-use parking lot. Restrooms, picnic facilities, lifeguard services, and telephones are available. Fee.

Camping

Tent and RV campsites are available Doheny State Beach. For camping reservations, call ParkNet (800) 444-7275.

Hazards

Extremely choppy seas and strong currents can be encountered during the afternoon on the west side of Dana Point. Be cautious when rounding Dana Point and avoid reefs and offshore rocks. Strong Santa Ana winds can occur at any time of the year. Always be prepared for the possibility of fog. Boat

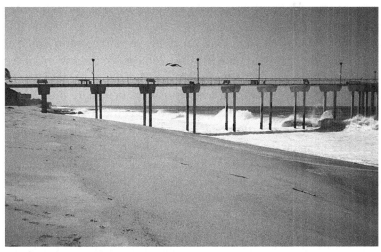

Large waves under Aliso Pier

traffic can be congested at the mouth of Dana Point Harbor; follow the rules of the road at all times.

Public access

Public beach access between Aliso Beach and Three Arch Bay is limited. Salt Creek Beach, a long, sandy beach to the northwest of Dana Point is accessible to the public.

Kayak surfing

Good waves for kayak surfing can be found at Doheny State Beach and at Salt Creek Beach. Avoid designated swimming and surfing areas.

Launching

Launch from the sand beach adjacent to the pier at Aliso Beach County Park. A surf launch may be necessary. Avoid designated swimming areas. This site has a very hazardous shorebreak when the waves a large.

Tour description

From Aliso Beach, head southeast. The narrow, sand beach is interrupted by occasional rocky headlands extending as shallow reefs offshore. Watch carefully for breaking water. The bluff is steep, with a relatively narrow marine terrace backed by rolling hills partly developed with homes. Pacific Coast Highway/Highway 1 is atop the marine terrace.

About two miles southeast of the launch site is Three Arch Bay, a scenic cove with craggy bluffs, sea caves, and rock arches. Landing is possible but the bluff top is privately owned and inaccessible to the public. Tide pools are abundant and filled with marine life. The beach and offshore waters have been designated as the South Laguna Marine Life Refuge, and taking of plants or animals is prohibited.

Southeast of Three Arch Bay is Salt Creek Beach, a long, sand beach extending to the west side of Dana Point. The beach faces southwest and is exposed to strong winds and waves. Seas during the afternoon can be very choppy. High on the bluff top overlooking the windswept beach are the private communities of Monarch Bay and Ritz Cove as well as the Ritz Carlton Hotel.

Directly ahead is Dana Point, a massive rocky headland named after Richard Henry Dana, Jr. In his book Two *Years Before the Mast*, Dana described his impressions of the early California coast while aboard the brig *Pilgrim* in 1835. The *Pilgrim* carried goods manufactured in New England around South America's Cape Horn to be traded for hides and tallow produced at the California Missions.

Shallow reefs and shoals extend about 350 yards off Dana Point. San Juan Rock, about 10 feet high and 50 feet across, lies about 250 yards offshore.

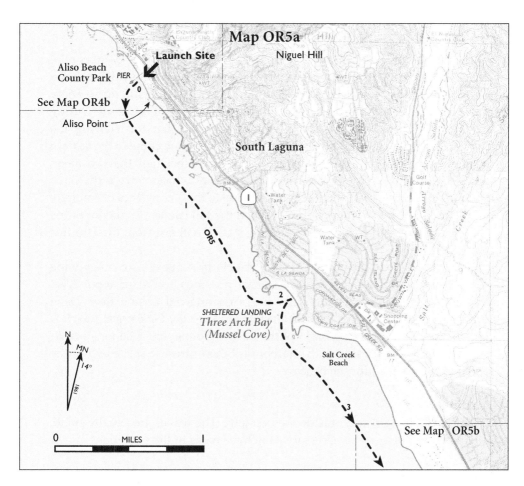

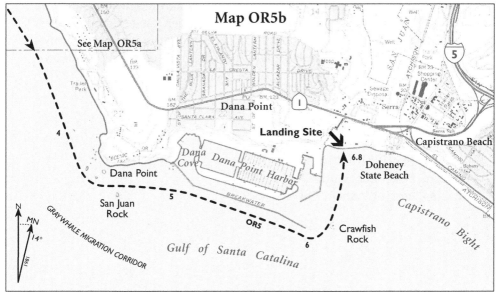

Trip OR5: Aliso Beach County Park to Doheny State Beach

Passage inside the rock is possible during calm conditions. The point is relatively flat-topped with high, steep bluffs. At low tide numerous tide pools are exposed along the rocky shoreline. Abundant marine life, including a variety of sea birds, sea lions, harbor seals, and dolphins is commonly seen. During winter and spring, Dana Point is an excellent location for viewing the California gray whales. Whales can be spotted when they come to the surface to breathe. The spout is a mist of condensed water, 10 feet high, that is exhaled under high pressure from the whale's lungs. Gray whales have a rhythmic breathing pattern. Usually they will make three to five short dives of a minute or less, followed by a long deep dive. When the tail (flukes) come out of the water, it usually signals a deep dive. A deep dive will last from three to five minutes.

On the east side of the point is Dana Point Harbor, an extensive man-made yacht harbor completed in 1971. The harbor provides berths for about 2,500 private yachts, a sport fishing fleet, and a commercial fishing fleet. Dana Harbor is headquarters for the official state tall-ship the *Californian*, which is moored in the west turning-basin of the harbor. Follow the mile-long breakwater along the south side of the harbor and then turn left at the end of the breakwater and head for the beach.

Landing

Land at Doheny Beach outside the east jetty. The waves are usually small, but a surf landing may be necessary. Watch for rocks in the surf zone.

What to do afterward

The visitor center at Doheny State Beach has aquariums, a simulated tide pool, and information about the Dana Point area. The Orange County Marine Institute, located at the west end of Dana Harbor, offers a variety of oceanographic classes. A replica of the square-rigged brig, the *Pilgrim*, is moored adjacent to the marine institute.

Alternate tour: OR1 or OR2

For more information

Doheny State Beach (714) 496-6172
Laguna Beach Lifeguards (714) 494-6571
Laguna Beach Weather (714) 494-6573

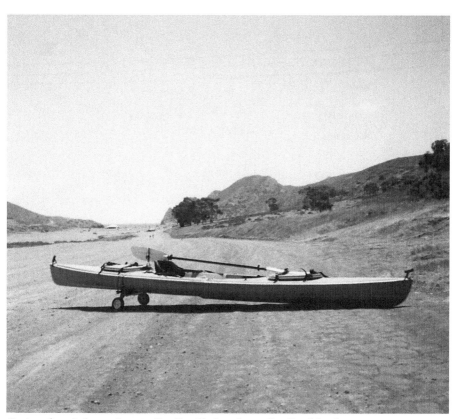

Portage from Isthmus Cove to Catalina Harbor, Santa Catalina Island

San Diego County Tours

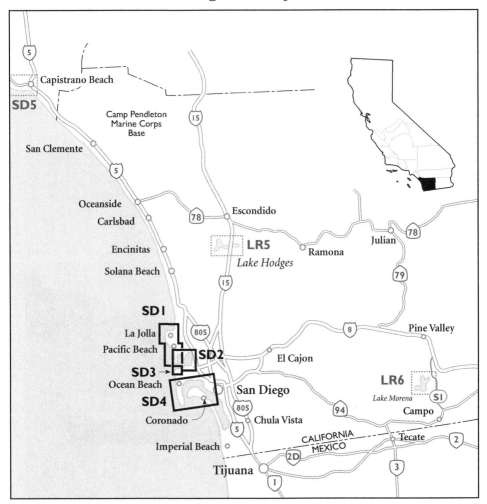

Tour		Skill Level	Length
SD1:	La Jolla Shores to Mission Bay	Intermediate	11.0 miles
SD2:	Mission Bay	Beginner	8.2 miles
SD3:	Dana Landing to Mission Bay Entrance	Beginner	3.5 miles
SD4:	San Diego Bay	Advanced	15.6 miles

Chapter 9

San Diego County

A low flying jet roared overhead. Helicopters were incessantly taking off and landing from the North Island Naval Air Station. Large and small naval vessels moved up and down the busy channel. Had World War III started? No, just an ordinary day in San Diego Bay. Earlier in the day I nearly had my video camera confiscated when a naval patrol boat found me shooting a video of a "sensitive area." I had no idea that the Point Loma Peninsula was sensitive but I guess they thought I was filming the nuclear submarines that were moored in the foreground. They warned me not to take any more videos but let me keep my film.

I breathed a sigh of relief when we finally passed Ballast Point and entered the natural area off Point Loma. The water in the lee of the point was calm and peaceful. A curious sea lion glanced at me as he hurriedly swam past, probably headed for the bait boats that we had passed a few moments before. We paddled close to shore, peering through the clear water at the waving strands of giant kelp. The Cabrillo Memorial high atop the peninsula was reflected in the glassy water.

At the head of the point, we paused for a lunch break before heading across the entrance channel to Coronado Island. There was a slight breeze coming from the west and the turquoise waves sparkled in the sunlight. A pod of dolphins paused briefly to ride the perfectly formed waves. I marveled at the gracefulness and ease with which they moved through the water. Moments later they were gone.

I turned around and gazed at the distant buildings of downtown San Diego silhouetted against the hazy sky. I could sense the pulsating energy of the busy metropolis. I felt so free and removed from the hustle and bustle of the city which was so near and yet so far away.

We finished our lunch and continued on our journey.

— San Diego Bay, September 20, 1996

TOUR SD1 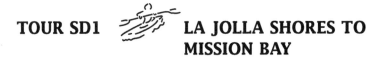 LA JOLLA SHORES TO MISSION BAY

Tour Details

Skill level:	Intermediate
Trip length/type:	11.0 miles; one-way; open-ocean; four to five hours
Chart/map:	NOAA Chart #18765; USGS *La Jolla* 7.5 min series

Summary

If fresh, salt air and the open ocean is your fancy, this paddle is for you. Along the way, explore the forests of giant kelp, gaze at the bottom through the clear water, play with the dolphins and sea lions, and pause to view the spectacular panorama of the San Diego coastline.

How to get there

To reach the launch site coming from the north, exit Interstate 5 at La Jolla Village Drive and go west to Torrey Pines Road. Go left on Torrey Pines Road to Ardath Drive and go right on Ardath Road to La Jolla Shores Drive. Go right on La Jolla Shores Drive to Avenida de la Playa. Go left on Avenida de la Playa to the beach. To reach the launch site coming from the south, exit Interstate 5 at Ardath Road and go west to La Jolla Shores Drive. Go right on La Jolla Shores Drive to Avenida de la Playa. Go left on Avenida de la Playa to the beach. Parking, restrooms, telephones, lifeguard services, and picnic facilities are available at Kellogg Park, about one block north of Avenida de la Playa. No fee.

To reach the landing site, exit Interstate 5 at Sea World Drive and go west about one mile to West Mission Bay Drive. Go right on West Mission Bay Drive/Ingraham Street, turn left off Ingraham Street onto to Dana Landing Road, and follow the signs to Dana Landing. Parking, restrooms, and telephones are available. No fee.

Camping

There are no public campgrounds in the immediate vicinity of the launch site. For information about the nearest state park campground, call ParkNet 1-800-444-7275.

Hazards

Avoid breaking and surging water when passing around Point La Jolla. Wear a helmet and PFD, and carry a waterproof flashlight when exploring the caves. Localized, thick kelp beds can make paddling difficult. Strong Santa Ana winds can occur any time of the year. Always be prepared for the possibility of fog. Boat traffic can be congested in Mission Bay; follow the rules of the road at all times.

Public access

The beach is accessible to the public along most of the route.

Kayak surfing

Good waves can be found at found at Marine Street Beach and Windansea Beach. Observe all posted swimming and board surfing areas.

Launching

Launch from the beach at La Jolla Shores. It is possible to drive onto the beach at Avenida de la Playa to unload your kayak. The waves are generally small, but a surf launch may be necessary.

Tour description

From the launch site head south toward the La Jolla cliffs. The water is usually clear and the white-sand bottom easily visible. La Jolla Canyon, a deep submarine canyon notched into the seafloor, lies about one thousand feet offshore. The area is a favorite place for scuba divers and has been protected as an underwater reserve encompassing 5,977 acres of tide and submerged lands. To the north lie Scripps Beach and Scripps Pier. On the hillside overlooking the beach is the Scripps Institute of Oceanography, one of the oldest and most best-known oceanographic research centers in the world.

As you approach the La Jolla cliffs watch for scuba divers. The wind and waves have eroded the sandstone cliffs, creating several sea caves. The name

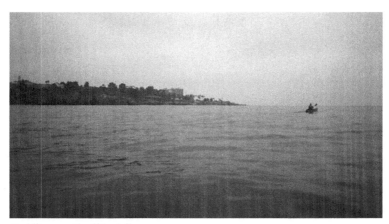

Paddling south off La Jolla

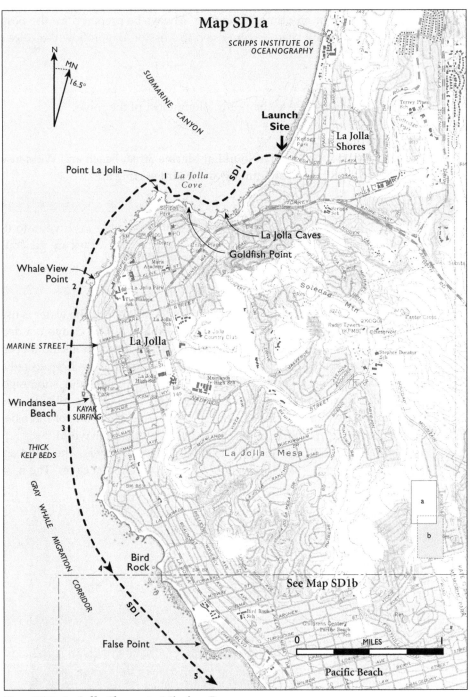

Map SD1a

SCRIPPS INSTITUTE OF
OCEANOGRAPHY

N
MN
16.5°

SUBMARINE CANYON

**Launch
Site**

La Jolla
Shores

Kellogg
Park

Point La Jolla

*La Jolla
Cove*

SD1

Scripps
Park

La Jolla Caves

Goldfish Point

Whale View
Point

2

Soledad Mtn

MARINE STREET

La Jolla

La Jolla
Country Club

Windansea
Beach

KAYAK
SURFING

3

THICK
KELP BEDS

La Jolla Mesa

GRAY WHALE MIGRATION CORRIDOR

4

Bird
Rock

See Map SD1b

a

b

0   MILES   1

False Point

Pacific Beach

5

Tour SD1: La Jolla Shores to Mission Bay

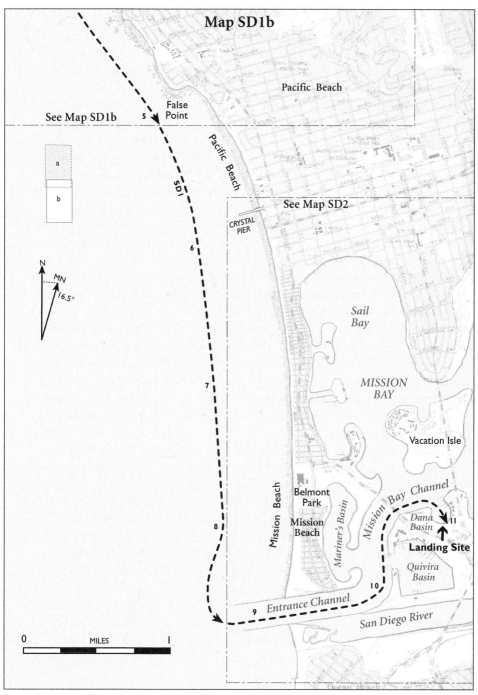

Map SD1b

Pacific Beach

See Map SD1b 5 → False Point

Pacific Beach

a

b

N
MN
16.5°

See Map SD2

CRYSTAL PIER

SD1

6

Sail Bay

MISSION BAY

7

Vacation Isle

8

Mission Beach

Belmont Park

Mission Beach

Mariner's Basin

Mission Bay Channel

Dana Basin

11

Landing Site

Quivira Basin

10

9 Entrance Channel

San Diego River

0   MILES   1

Tour SD1 (continued)

"La Jolla" was derived from the Spanish term for a cave in the bluff worn by waves. The best-known cave, at Gold Fish Point (named for the abundance of bright orange garibaldi in the area), can be explored at a medium-to-high tide on a calm day. The tide pools support a wide variety of sea life. Just inside Point La Jolla is La Jolla Cove, a sheltered cove noted for its water clarity and beautiful sand beach.

Approach Point La Jolla cautiously. Large swells can emerge suddenly from the deep water. South of the point are small pocket beaches separated by low, rocky headlands. Most of the beaches are accessible to the public. Beautiful homes are clustered along the shoreline. The beaches are popular and the waves are usually crowded with surfers. Windansea Beach, about one and one-half miles south of La Jolla Cove, is one of the more popular surfing spots in the San Diego area.

Offshore, a thick kelp forest provides the perfect habitat for a variety of fish and marine mammals. Harbor seals and sea lions are commonly seen year-round, and in the winter California gray whales pass close to shore. The kelp beds extend nearly a mile offshore and can make paddling difficult. Landing is possible in the sheltered coves, but watch carefully for submerged reefs and be prepared for a strong shore break.

At False Point, about four miles south of Point La Jolla, the rocky bluffs of the La Jolla shoreline discontinue. To the south are the wide sand beaches of Pacific Beach and Mission Beach. Tourmaline Surfing Park, on the south side of False Point is a favorite surfing spot. Crystal Pier, about one mile south of False Point, was constructed in 1926 to attract land buyers to the area. The pier contained shops, arcades, and a ballroom. In 1936 the pier was remodeled with a motel and cottages. It is supposedly the only pier on the West Coast which provides lodging. South of Crystal Pier is Mission Beach Park, also known as the Belmont Park. A huge roller coaster, the Giant Dipper, can be seen from the water. The coaster was first opened in 1925, and in 1975 was declared a State Historical Landmark. Mission Beach and Pacific Beach are crowded with swimmers and surfers, and landing is not recommended.

Watch for surging waves at the entrance to Mission Bay. Stay on the right side of the Entrance Channel and avoid fishing lines coming off the jetty. Watch carefully for emerging boats when crossing the side-channel to Quivira Basin.

Landing
Land at the launch ramp at Dana Basin.

What to do afterward
Belmont Park is located in nearby Mission Beach.

Alternate tour: SD2

For more information
San Diego Parks and Recreation, Coastal Parks Division (619) 221-8901
San Diego Lifeguards (619) 221-8899
San Diego Weather (619) 221-8884

TOUR SD2 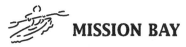 MISSION BAY

Tour Details

Skill level:	Beginner
Trip length/type:	8.2 miles; round-trip; bay; three to four hours
Chart/map:	NOAA Chart #s 18740 and 18765; USGS *La Jolla* 7.5 min series

Summary

On this round-trip excursion of Mission Bay you will visit calm, sandy lagoons, the San Diego Aquatic Center, two wildlife reserves, the Mission Bay Visitor Center and Sea World.

How to get there

To reach the launch site, exit Interstate 5 at Sea World Drive and proceed west about one mile to West Mission Bay Drive. Go right on West Mission Bay Drive/Ingraham Street, turn left off Ingraham Street onto to Dana Landing Road, and follow the signs to Dana Landing. Parking, restrooms, and telephones are available. No fee.

Camping

Camping is available at the Campland on the Bay. For reservations call (800) 422-9386.

Hazards

This tour is entirely within Mission Bay. Boat traffic can be congested; follow the rules of the road at all times. Be particularly cautious of high-speed crafts such as jet skis and water-ski boats. Avoid posted swimming areas and be alert when passing water-ski launch sites. Avoid fishing lines when paddling near docks or jetties. Gusty winds and choppy conditions are likely to be encountered during the afternoon. Fog can occur at any time of the year. If possible plan your trip route to have a following tidal current.

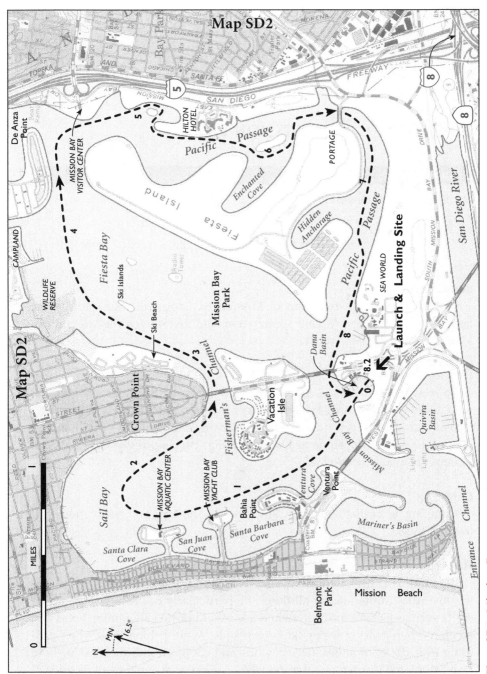

Tour SD2: Mission Bay

Public access
Public access to the water is available throughout most of Mission Bay.

Launching
Launch from the paved boat ramp at Dana Landing.

Tour description
From Dana Basin head northwest across Mission Bay Channel toward Ventura Point. Watch for boating traffic when crossing the channel. The West Mission Bay Drive bridge is on the left and the Ingraham Street bridge is on the right. Stay to the west side of the channel as you pass Ventura Point. North of the point is Ventura Cove, a sheltered inlet with a sand beach and good swimming. Boat speed is limited to five knots, keeping wakes at a minimum. From Ventura Cove, continue to paddle north. Condominiums and a hotel are clustered along the narrow sand beach at Bahia Point, creating a resort atmosphere. Located on the narrow sliver of land separating Santa Barbara and San Juan coves is the Mission Bay Yacht Club. To the east, across Sail Bay is Fisherman's Channel, which leads to Fiesta Bay.

From the Mission Bay Yacht Club continue north across the entrance to San Juan Cove to the Mission Bay Aquatic Center. The Aquatic Center is the world's largest instructional and recreational waterfront aquatic facility. The center was established in 1971 as a cooperative collegiate facility for the use of students, faculty, staff, and alumni of all San Diego County colleges, universities, and youth organizations. The facility offers instructional and recreational opportunities in water skiing, sailing, surfing, rowing, kayaking, scuba diving and wind surfing.

From Santa Clara Point head east across Sail Bay. Conditions can become choppy during the afternoon, but fortunately the wind should be coming from astern. Pass beneath the Ingraham Street bridge into Fiesta Bay and head north along Crown Point. The beach on the east side of Crown Point is sheltered from the westerly wind and there are picnic facilities, fire rings, and restrooms. Fiesta Bay is an open-speed area, so be alert for jet skis and water skiers. Observe the posted rules when crossing water-ski landing and take-off zones.

Two wildlife reserves, the Northern Wildlife Reserve (an 88-acre salt marsh/mud flat complex) and the 21-acre Kendall-Frost Marsh are located at the north end of Fiesta Bay. The Northern Wildlife Reserve is owned by the City of San Diego and the Kendall-Frost Marsh is part of the University of California Natural Reserve System. These two preserves are the only remaining natural wildlife habitats within Mission Bay City Park. Boating is prohibited within the reserves.

Mission Bay was known by early explorers as *Bahia Falsa* (False Bay) because it was often mistaken as the entrance to San Diego Bay. Formed by the San Diego River delta, the bay was a maze of mud flats, shallow marshes, and channels which provided a primary feeding and nesting habitat for a large variety of migratory and resident birds. In the early 1960s the river was channelized and the bay was dredged and modified to its current configuration. Despite the changes, several species of birds including the endangered California least tern continue to nest and breed in the reserves. Other birds commonly seen include grebes, snowy egrets, blue herons, loons, teals, and gulls. Campland, a private campground facility, and the De Anza Harbor Resort are east of the marshland.

From the De Anza Resort head south, following the Pacific Passage, a narrow waterway separating Fiesta Island from the mainland. On the left bank is the Mission Bay Visitor Center. The grounds are nicely landscaped and facilities include picnic areas, paved walking and bike paths, restrooms, a snack bar, a physical fitness course, and a basketball court. Fiesta Island is mostly undeveloped and is used as a launch site for jet skis and water skiers. A one-way road circles the island providing access to the beach. The mud flats of the island provide a habitat for several species of shorebirds including the ruddy turnstone, willet, and black-bellied plover.

South of the visitor center are several scenic lagoons and the Hilton Hotel. The beach in front of the hotel is a popular site for wind surfing. About one mile south of the Hilton is the causeway to Fiesta Island. Land on the Fiesta Island side of the causeway and portage the short distance across the road, watching carefully for cars. South of the causeway continue to follow the Pacific Passage, which turns west. This is a designated jet ski area, so be sure to follow the posted warnings. During the afternoon a headwind may be encountered on this leg of the voyage.

To the west of the jet ski area is Sea World, a 130-acre marine park with educational exhibits, marine shows, and aquariums. Follow closely along the shoreline to capture the sights and sounds of this world-famous marine park. Free entertainment is provided by local pelicans, gulls, occasional sea lions, and a group of Sea World penguins housed in a pen along the bank of the bay. At the west end of Sea World is an aerial tram and a huge open-air arena for the marine shows. Keep your distance from the facility to avoid disturbing the animals. After passing beneath the Ingraham Street bridge head south into Dana Basin.

Landing
Land at the launch ramp at Dana Basin where you launched.

What to do afterward

Sea World is located across the street from Dana Landing. Old Town San Diego State Historic Park, a re-creation of early California lifestyle, is off Interstate 5 about two miles southeast of Mission Bay. Mission San Diego de Alcala is about five miles east of Mission Bay.

Alternate tour: LR5

For more information

San Diego Parks and Recreation, Coastal Parks Division (619) 221-8901
San Diego Lifeguards (619) 221-8899
San Diego Weather (619) 221-8884

TOUR SD3 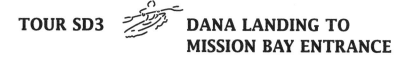 DANA LANDING TO MISSION BAY ENTRANCE

Tour Details	
Skill level:	Beginner
Trip length/type:	3.5 miles; round-trip; bay; one to two hours
Chart/map:	NOAA Chart #s 18740 and 18765; USGS *La Jolla* 7.5 min series

Summary

Easy access from downtown San Diego makes this trip the perfect "wind down" cruise following a hard day at the office or when you just want a quick get-away. Breathe the fresh air and capture the moment as you meander through the bay and watch the beautiful sunset. Along the way you'll see lots of pelicans, gulls, cormorants, and perhaps even a sea lion or a harbor seal looking for a handout.

How to get there

To reach the launch site, exit Interstate 5 at Sea World Drive and proceed west about one mile to West Mission Bay Drive. Go right on West Mission Bay Drive/Ingraham Street, turn left off Ingraham Street onto to Dana Landing Road, and follow the signs to Dana Landing. Parking, restrooms, and telephones are available. No fee.

Camping

Camping is available at the Campland on the Bay. For reservations call (800) 422-9386.

Hazards

This tour is entirely within Mission Bay. Boat traffic can be congested; follow the rules of the road at all times. Avoid fishing lines when paddling near docks or jetties. Choppy conditions can develop in the Entrance Channel during the afternoon, and winter storms can create hazardous waves at the harbor mouth. Fog can occur any time of the year. Check your tide book before departing and plan your trip to take advantage of the tidal flow.

Public access

Public access to the water is available throughout most of Mission Bay.

Kayak surfing

Waves for kayak surfing can be found outside the harbor entrance.

Launching

Launch from the paved boat ramp at Dana Landing.

Tour description

From Dana Basin, enter the Mission Bay Channel and head west. Pass beneath the West Mission Bay Drive bridge, then cross to the west side of the channel. At Mission Point the channel turns west. Stay to the right side of the Entrance Channel and watch out for fishing lines from anglers on the jetty. Surge and wind chop may increase in size as you approach the harbor mouth. If you enjoy kayak surfing, good waves can be found outside the jetties. During the winter, beware of large storm swells that occasionally break across the harbor mouth. Pause for a few moments breathing the fresh salty air and watch the sun slowly sink into the sea.

Carefully cross to the south side of the Entrance Channel and follow the jetty back toward the bay. At the east end of the Entrance Channel the jetty makes a sharp turn north. Just past the bend, enter Quivira Basin, making a 180 degree turn, then follow the west side of the basin past the harbor offices. Continue counterclockwise around the perimeter of the basin, meandering through the maze of boats, piers, and docks. The air is cool and still and the evening harbor lights dance across the smooth water. Re-enter the main channel and return to Dana Basin.

Landing

Land at the launch ramp at Dana Basin where you launched.

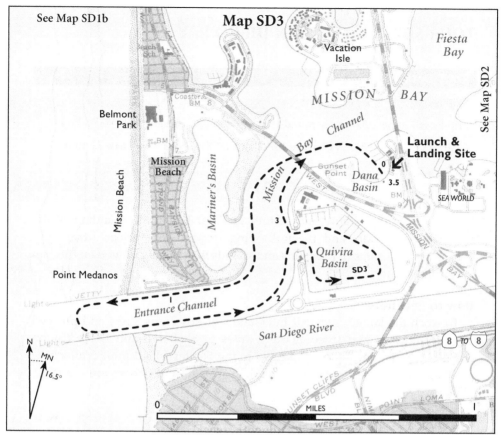

Tour SD3: Dana Landing to Mission Bay Entrance

What to do afterward

After your paddle, enjoy an evening with friends at one of Mission Bay's fine restaurants.

Alternate tour: LR5

For more information

San Diego Parks and Recreation, Coastal Parks Division (619) 221-8901
San Diego Lifeguards (619) 221-8899
San Diego Weather (619) 221-8884

TOUR SD4 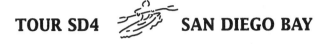 SAN DIEGO BAY

Tour Details

Skill level:	Advanced
Trip length/type:	15.6 miles; round-trip; bay and open-ocean; six to seven hours
Chart/map:	NOAA Chart #s 18772 and 18773; USGS *Point Loma* 7.5 min series

Summary

The captivating beauty and history of Point Loma, the grandeur of the Hotel del Coronado, and the forbidding presence of nuclear attack submarines are just some of the sights and sounds that will engulf you on this San Diego adventure.

How to get there

To reach the launch site, exit Interstate 5 at Rosecrans Street and proceed south about two and three-quarters miles to Shelter Island Drive (Byron Street). Turn left and follow the signs to the Shelter Island public launching ramp at the northeast end of the island. Restrooms and phones are available. No fee.

Camping

There are no public campgrounds in the immediate vicinity of the launch site. For information about the nearest state park campground, call ParkNet (800) 444-7275.

Hazards

Strong, gusty wind and choppy conditions are common both inside and outside the harbor during the afternoon. Hazardous seas may be encountered outside the harbor during a south or a northwest swell. Boat traffic can be congested; follow the rules of the road at all times. Shallow reefs extend off Point Loma and at Zuniga Shoal. Avoid all breaking and surging waves at both these locations. Strong Santa Ana winds can occur at any time of the year. Always be prepared for the possibility of fog. Check your tide book before departing and plan your trip to take advantage of the tidal flow.

Public access

Numerous public launch sites are available on Coronado Island and in San Diego Bay, but entry and landing are prohibited on military reservations. Observe all posted warnings.

Kayak surfing

Good waves for kayak surfing can be found off Point Loma.

Launching

Launch from the paved launch ramp near the northeast end of Shelter Island.

Tour description

From the launch ramp head southwest, staying between the shoreline and the boats anchored just offshore. To the east, the tall buildings of downtown San Diego rise above San Diego bay. To the southeast across the main channel is Coronado Island, and to the west are the hills of the Point Loma Peninsula

At approximately one mile you will reach the southwest end of the Shelter Island. Carefully cross the Shelter Island Channel to the Point Loma Peninsula. To your right is La Playa, a narrow, sandy beach. Known as "Hide Park," La Playa was the West Coast's most successful hide-tanning operation between 1824 and 1846. Straight ahead is the United States Naval Research and Development Facility (NRD). Some of the vessels anchored at the NRD look more like spacecraft than boats. It may sound strange to hear sea lions barking in this setting, but look carefully and you will see the floating pens used to house sea lions and other marine mammals which are trained for military purposes. Stay well offshore; this is a restricted military area.

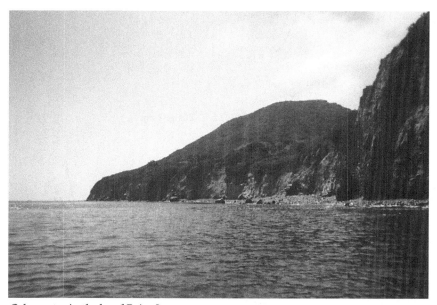

Calm water in the lee of Point Loma

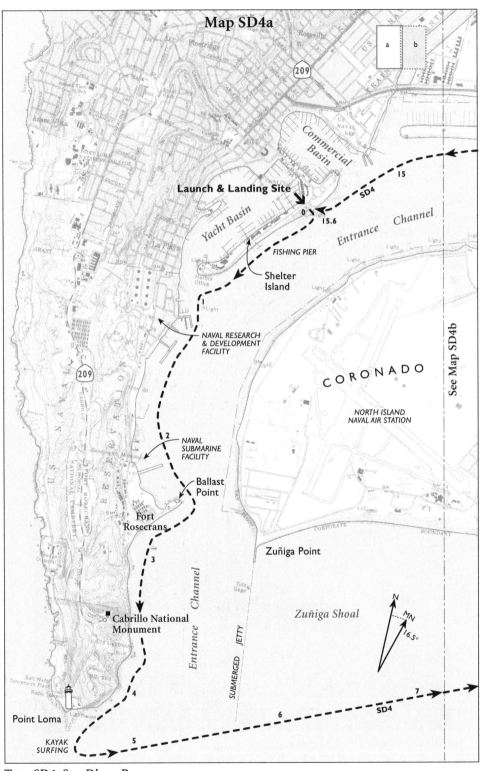

Map SD4a

Commercial Basin

209

Launch & Landing Site

Yacht Basin

SD4

15

0

15.6

Entrance Channel

FISHING PIER

Shelter
Island

Light

Light

Light

Light

Harbor Office

Light

NAVAL RESEARCH
& DEVELOPMENT
FACILITY

CORONADO

See Map SD4b

209

NORTH ISLAND
NAVAL AIR STATION

2

NAVAL
SUBMARINE
FACILITY

Ballast
Point

Fort
Rosecrans

Zuñiga Point

3

Entrance Channel

Zuñiga Shoal

N

MN

16.5°

Cabrillo National
Monument

Tide Gage

SUBMERGED JETTY

7

SD4

Point Loma

KAYAK
SURFING

4

5

6

Tour SD4: San Diego Bay

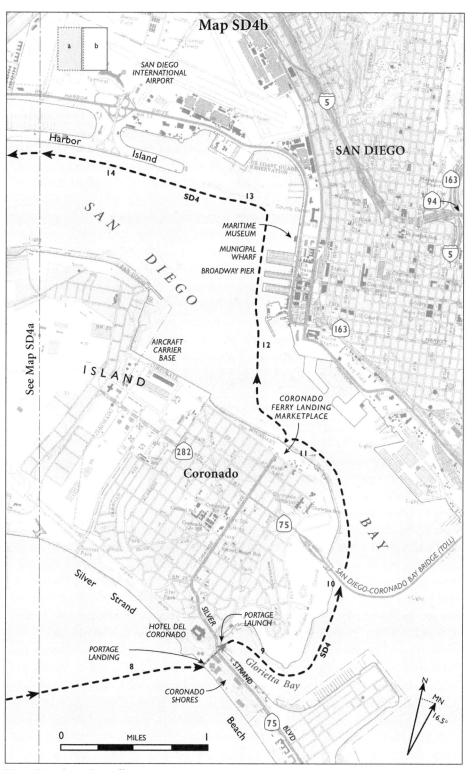

Map SD4b

a   b

SAN DIEGO
INTERNATIONAL
AIRPORT

5

SAN DIEGO

163

Harbor

94

Island

14

5

SD4

13

MARITIME
MUSEUM

MUNICIPAL
WHARF

BROADWAY PIER

163

S
A
N

D
I
E
G
O

AIRCRAFT
CARRIER
BASE

12

ISLAND

CORONADO
FERRY LANDING
MARKETPLACE

See Map SD4a

282

11

Coronado

75

B
A
Y

SAN DIEGO-CORONADO BAY BRIDGE (TOLL)

10

Silver

SD4

Strand

SILVER

PORTAGE
LAUNCH

HOTEL DEL
CORONADO

9

PORTAGE
LANDING

STRAND

Glorietta Bay

8

CORONADO
SHORES

N

Beach

75

BLVD

MN
16.5°

0   MILES   1

Tour SD4 (continued)

From the NRD continue southwest. On the right, several bait barges lie at anchor. The barges are alive with activity as thousands of pelicans and gulls swarm overhead and playful sea lions thrash about in the water looking for a handout. In stark contrast are the ominous nuclear submarines tied to the docks at the Naval Submarine Facility. Keep your distance from these metallic predators of the deep sea.

Approximately one and one-half miles south of Shelter Island is Ballast Point. Rounded cobbles found on the point were used as ballast in days past. Today, a Coast Guard station and pier occupy the end of the point. South of Ballast Point is Point Loma, a scenic natural area rivaling any on the California coast. High sandstone cliffs vegetated with coastal sage scrub overlook the calm waters in the lee of the point. The Cabrillo National Monument, built in commemoration of Juan Rodriguez Cabrillo, who discovered San Diego in 1542, stands atop the narrow headland. The memorial includes a visitor center, exhibit hall, auditorium, gift shop, and scenic overlook. A one and one-half mile trail winds along the top of the bluff.

Approach Point Loma cautiously. A shallow reef extending south of the point causes the waves to break well offshore. Numerous shipwrecks, littering the seafloor, attest to the perilous conditions. If you are skilled at kayak surfing and prepared to get wet, try the waves at Ralph's, a well-known surfing spot on the point.

The original lighthouse on Point Loma was constructed in 1854. Built of sandstone and brick, it is one of the first New England-style light houses on the West Coast. The original lighthouse was built high on the bluff, and because its oil-lamp beacon was often obscured during heavy fog, a new, more visible lighthouse was constructed at a lower elevation in 1891.

From Point Loma head northeast across the Entrance Channel to San Diego Bay. Watch carefully for approaching ships when crossing the channel. To the east of the channel is Zuniga Shoal and a submerged rock jetty. A lighted beacon and foghorn mark the south end of the reef. Avoid all breaking and surging water when crossing the shoal. To the east, on Coronado Island, is a distinct group of tall buildings (Coronado Shores). Set a course just to the left of the buildings. If visibility is poor or you would prefer to paddle closer to shore, paddle north to the beach (after passing Zuniga Shoal) and follow the Coronado Island shoreline southeast until you reach the tall buildings.

As you approach the Coronado Shores buildings, the Hotel del Coronado, with its distinctive red-domed roof, should be visible to the left of the buildings. Land on the sand beach between the Hotel del Coronado and the Coronado Shores. A convenient place to portage across Coronado Island to Glorietta Bay is at Avenida del Sol, a short street that runs between the Hotel del Coronado parking lot and the Coronado Shores. Cross Silver Strand Boulevard at the crosswalk in front of the Hotel del Coronado. Directly across

Silver Strand Boulevard from Avenida del Sol is the Hotel del Coronado's old boathouse, which has been converted to a Chart House restaurant. Launch from the narrow sand beach just west of the restaurant. If time allows, a quick tour through the Hotel del Coronado is well worthwhile (even in your bathing suit). The old hotel, constructed in 1887, is the largest wooden Victorian building in California.

From Glorietta Bay, follow the Coronado shoreline north toward the San Diego-Coronado Bay Bridge. San Diego Bay extends another five miles southeast to Imperial Beach. The San Diego-Coronado Bay Bridge was constructed in 1969 to replace the old Coronado ferry service. The bridge has an interesting curved shape resembling part of a roller coaster at an amusement park. The bridge is 246 feet high at its highest point. Pause for a few moments beneath the bridge and listen to the continuous rumbling of traffic passing overhead.

About one mile northwest of the San Diego-Coronado Bay Bridge is the Coronado Ferry-Landing Marketplace, a pleasant rest stop with shops, a delicatessen, and a restaurant. A sand beach allows for easy access. Across the bay is downtown San Diego with its tall buildings.

From the marketplace, cross the bay to the San Diego waterfront. Seaport Village, the site of the Old Coronado Ferry Landing on the San Diego side, consists of 22 acres of park lands, shops, restaurants, and galleries. To the north of Seaport Village is G Street Pier, a popular fishing spot, and Broadway Pier, a good place from which to view the bay and downtown. The San Diego Maritime Museum is home to three historic ships: the *Star of India*, the *Medea*, and the *Berkeley*. The three ships have been beautifully restored and now house various museum exhibits. Tours are offered daily.

From the Maritime Museum head west past Harbor Island. The bay is very wide at this point and shipping traffic should not be a hazard. During the afternoon a strong headwind may be encountered and conditions may be choppy. Across the channel on Coronado Island is the North Island Naval Air Station. Moored along the quay at North Island are the formidable aircraft carriers, the largest ships in the US Navy. In 1927 Charles Lindbergh began his famous transatlantic flight form North Island. Today North Island Naval Air Station is home to all carrier-based anti-submarine warfare squadrons.

As you approach Shelter Island the wind and chop should begin to diminish. On the right is the Commercial Basin, home of the commercial fishing fleet. Be careful to avoid boating traffic when crossing the entrance to the basin.

Landing
Land at the paved launch ramp at the northeast end of Shelter Island where you launched.

What to do afterward

The Cabrillo National Monument and Old Point Loma lighthouse are at the end of Catalina Boulevard on Point Loma. Shelter Island has several nice restaurants.

Alternate tour: SD2 or SD3

For more information

San Diego Parks and Recreation, Coastal Parks Division (619) 221-8901
San Diego Lifeguards (619) 221-8899
San Diego Weather (619) 221-8884

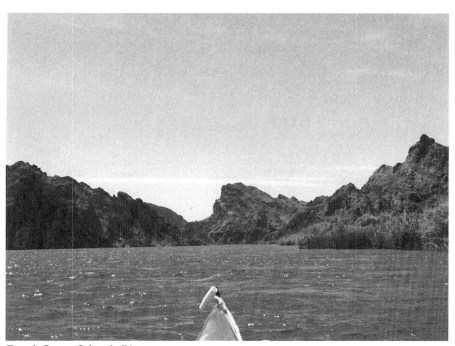

Topock Gorge, Colorado River

Lake & River Tours

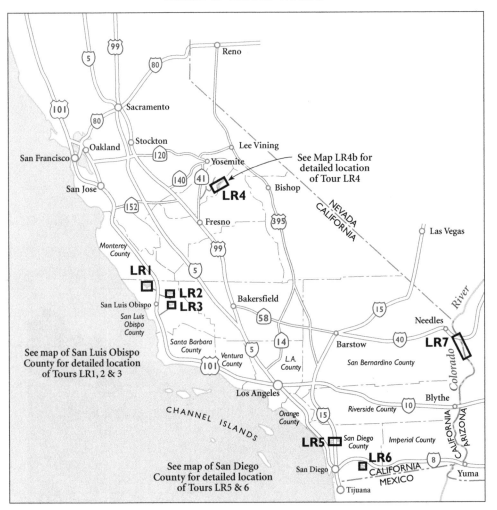

Tour	Skill Level	Length
LR1: Lake Nacimiento, San Luis Obispo County	Intermediate	16.5 miles
LR2: Santa Margarita Lake, San Luis Obispo County	Beginner	12.4 miles
LR3: Lopez Lake, San Luis Obisbo County	Beginner	14.3 miles
LR4: Mammoth Pool Reservoir, Fresno/ Madera Cos.	Beginner	12.5 miles
LR5: Lake Hodges, San Diego County	Beginner	14.0 miles
LR6: Lake Morena, San Diego County	Beginner	8.5 miles
LR7: Topock Gorge, San Bernadino County	Beginner	16.6 miles

Chapter 10

Lakes and Rivers

It was spring in the Santa Lucia Mountains. The hills were green and the flowers were in full bloom. We'd had a rainy winter so the lake was very full. I like to paddle lakes during the winter and spring when its too stormy to paddle in the ocean and the lakes are at full capacity.

It was a calm day during mid-week, and there were only a few boats on the lake. There weren't any water skiers or jet skis—which I didn't miss. I was enjoying the peace and quiet and taking my time.

I had been on the water for about an hour and had already seen some deer grazing along the shore and what I thought was an eagle soaring high overhead. It's always fun to paddle in a lake because you get to see a whole different variety of plants and animals than you see in the ocean. I stopped to video a sign, which marked a restricted speed area, when I noticed something moving in the background on the shore. At first it didn't really catch my attention but when it moved again I turned the camera and zoomed in on the object. My jaw dropped when I saw a large cat walking slowly down to the edge of the lake. At first I thought it was a mountain lion but after I steadied the camera and got a better look, I realized it was a lynx. The long, lanky cat had brown fur, with a relatively short tail and tufted ears. I was only a short distance away and he hadn't seen me. I had seen bobcats and black bears in the wild but never a large cat. I kept the video focused on the animal as he walked to the edge of the lake for a drink of water.

He lapped the water for a few minutes then slowly walked back up the hill, rubbing the bushes and scratching the ground as he went. I watched him disappear into the trees.

— Lake Nacimiento, March 14, 1997

TOUR LR1   LAKE NACIMIENTO, SAN LUIS OBISPO COUNTY

Tour Details

Skill level:	Intermediate
Trip length/type:	16.5 miles; round-trip; five to six hours
Chart/map:	Maps are available at the park entrance; USGS *Lime Mountain* and *Tierra Redondo Mountain* 7.5 min series

Summary

165 miles of pristine shoreline surround this scenic lake located halfway between San Francisco and Los Angeles. As you meander along the forested shoreline you're likely to see deer or perhaps a bobcat or an eagle. The lake is open daily. Swimming is permitted.

How to get there

To reach Lake Nacimiento, exit Highway 101 at Highway 46 in Paso Robles. Go west on 24th Street to Nacimiento Lake Drive (County Road G-14). Continue west on Nacimiento Lake Drive for 16 miles to the Lake Nacimiento Resort entrance. Park in the lot adjacent to the launch ramp at the resort. Restrooms, picnic facilities, phones, and a store, are provided. Fee.

Camping

Tent and RV campsites are available at the Lake Nacimiento Resort. For reservations call (800) 323-3839.

Hazards

Hot weather, strong gusty winds, boat traffic, submerged rocks and snags, rattlesnakes, ticks, and poison oak are all possible hazards. The surface area of the lake fluctuates with varying water level. Be sure to call ahead for current lake level. This tour describes conditions at a relatively high water level.

Public access

Most of the lake shoreline is privately owned. Check with the park ranger for day-use landing areas.

Kayak surfing

None

Launching

Launch from the beach or the launch ramp at the resort. The floating dock is useful for loading gear. Another public boat ramp is available at the North Shore day-use area on the north side of Nacimiento Dam. Be courteous to other boaters by moving quickly away from the ramp after launching.

Tour description

Nacimiento means "special birth place" in the Chumash language. Construction of the Nacimiento Dam began in 1956, and the reservoir was filled in 1959. When full, the lake is 18 miles long, with 165 miles of shoreline. Total capacity of the lake is 350,000 acre feet. It is used primarily for irrigation and flood control for the Salinas Valley. The lake is noted for its great white bass fishing, its calm winds, and an average water temperature of 72 degrees, perfect for swimming and water skiing.

The main body of the lake is oriented in an east-west direction with most of the tributaries entering the lake at right angles. The headwaters are located at the west end of the lake, the dam at the east end. The primary water source is the Nacimiento River, which enters the lake from the west. Lake Nacimiento Resort is on the south shore near the dam. Most of the shoreline at the west end is privately owned, and landing is prohibited. Limited day-use landing is permitted along Monterey County-owned shoreline at the east end of the lake. Overnight camping is permitted only in designated campgrounds.

From the launch ramp at the marina, cross the lake and head south. Stay to the right of the centerline buoys when paddling in the main channel. At about one mile, you will round a broad, low-lying headland and head west. The shoreline is rocky with numerous small coves and bays. In the morning and evening, deer can often be seen grazing on the grasslands overlooking the lake.

At two and one-half miles you will reach Bee Rock, a prominent rock outcropping on the north shore. Just beyond is Bee Rock Cove, a private development with numerous residences. West of Bee Rock, the lake narrows and turns sharply left. Just west of the bend is Las Tablas Arm, a large embayment on the south shore. Carefully cross the main channel of the lake, observing the rules of the road, and enter the Las Tablas Arm. Several private residential developments are located on the western shore. The eastern shore is accessible to the public for day-use.

Continue along the west shore of Las Tablas Arm for about one mile to Town Creek, a narrow tributary entering the lake from the west. A white, five-MPH buoy marks the entrance. After a sharp switchback turn, you will enter a narrow canyon with steep banks. The south side of the canyon is vegetated with oaks and pines while the north side is vegetated with chaparral and sage. The air is usually still and warm and the water calm and glassy. Insects dance across the water and an occasional fish can be seen breaking the smooth

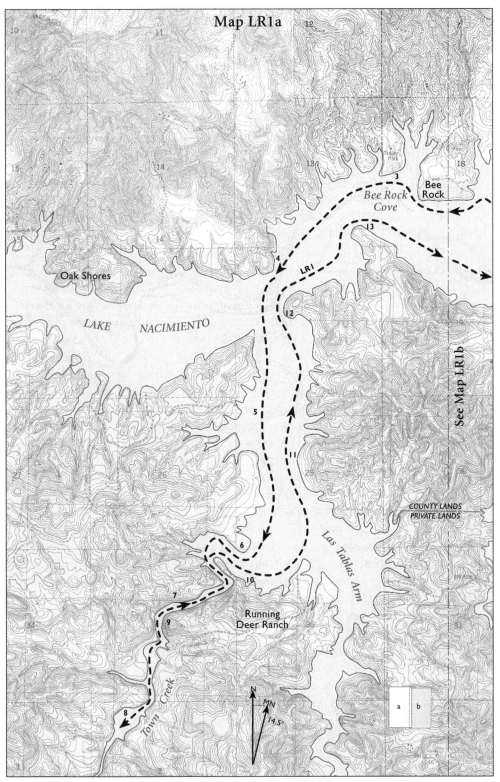

Map LR1a

Bee Rock Cove

Bee Rock

Oak Shores

LAKE   NACIMIENTO

LR1

See Map LR1b

COUNTY LANDS
PRIVATE LANDS

Las Tablas Arm

Running
Deer Ranch

Town Creek

N
MN
14.5°

a   b

Tour LR1: Lake Nacimiento, San Luis Obispo County

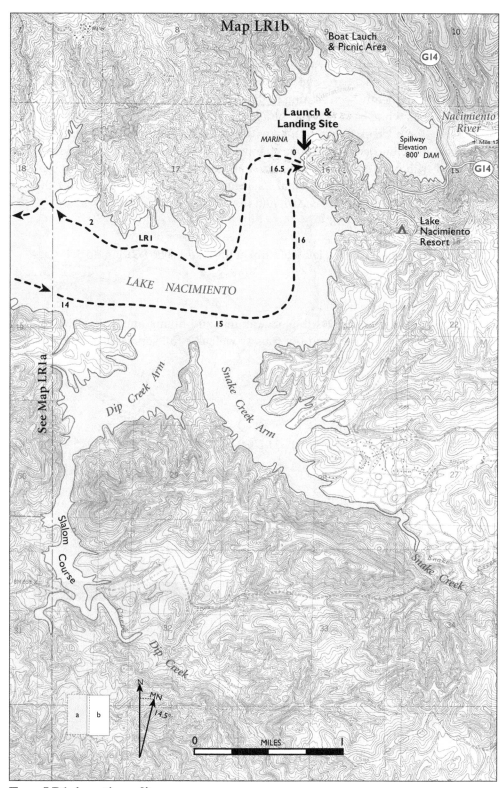

Tour LR1 (continued)

surface. After a sharp turn west, the canyon opens into a valley with oaks and grasslands. There are a few cabins along the shoreline and wildlife is abundant. Bobcats, black bears, and even mountain lions roam this territory and eagles are frequently seen soaring high overhead. If you happen to have your fishing pole, white bass, crappie, bluegill and catfish are plentiful.

From Town Creek return to the Las Tablas Arm. Cross the bay and follow the east shoreline back to the main channel of the lake. The grassy hillsides are shaded with oaks and pines. Head east at the main channel and follow centerline buoys back to the marina. Landing is permitted along most of the shoreline between Las Tablas Arm and the marina.

Landing
Land at the beach or the launch ramp at the resort. The floating dock is useful for unloading gear.

What to do afterward
Fishing, water skiing, boating, swimming, and hiking are available at the resort. A swimming pool and hot tubs as well as a full-service restaurant are open during the summer.

Alternate tour: LR2

For more information
Lake Nacimiento Resort (800) 323-3839
Lake Patrol (805) 238-2376

TOUR LR2   SANTA MARGARITA LAKE, SAN LUIS OBISPO COUNTY

Tour Details	
Skill level:	Beginner
Trip length/type:	12.4 miles; round-trip; three to four hours
Chart/map:	Maps are available at the park entrance; USGS *Santa Margarita Lake* 7.5 min series

Summary
Mountain lions and bears roam the hills surrounding this obscure lake in eastern San Luis Obispo County. Along the route you will stop at several

locations to observe the unique fauna and flora indigenous to the area. The lake is open daily. Swimming is not permitted.

How to get there

To reach Santa Margarita Lake Regional Park exit Highway 101 at Highway 58 between San Luis Obispo and Atascadero. Go east approximately three miles, through the town of Santa Margarita, and turn right on Pozo Road. Follow Pozo Road for about six miles, then turn left on Lake Road and proceed to the park entrance. Park in the parking lot at White Oak Flat. Restrooms, picnic facilities, phones, a store, and a launch ramp are provided. Fee.

Camping

Tent and RV campsites are available the Santa Margarita Lake Regional Park. For group reservations call (805) 781-5219.

Hazards

Hot weather, strong gusty winds, boat traffic, submerged rocks and snags, rattlesnakes, ticks, and poison oak are all possible hazards. The surface area of the lake fluctuates with varying water level. Be sure to call ahead for current lake level. This tour describes conditions at a relatively high water level.

Public access

The entire shoreline of the lake is within Santa Margarita Lake Regional Park and is accessible to the public.

Kayak surfing

None

Launching

Launch from the beach or the launch ramp at White Oak Flat. A floating dock is available for loading gear. Be courteous to other boaters by moving quickly away from the ramp after launching.

Tour description

The Salinas Dam was constructed during World War II to provide water for Camp San Luis Obispo. Today Santa Margarita Lake is a major source of drinking water for the city of San Luis Obispo. The main body of the lake is oriented in an east-west, with most of the tributaries entering the lake from the north or south. The primary source of water for the lake is the Salinas River, which flows in from the east. The dam is at the west end, and the park concessions are on the south shore. The primitive Sapwi Boat Camp is on the

Map LR2

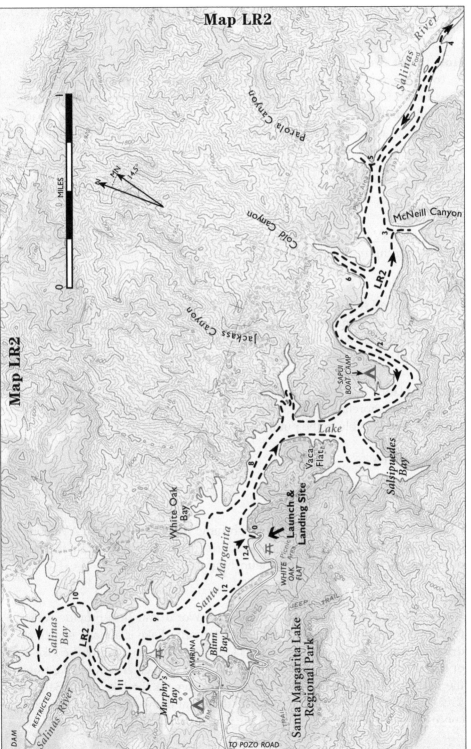

north shore across from Salsipuedes Bay. Surrounding the lake are several thousand acres of designated open space and within the open space are 25 miles of trails available to hikers, bicyclists, and equestrians.

From the launch ramp at White Oak Flat head east, following the shoreline counterclockwise. On the right is Vaca Flat, a day-use area with picnic tables, barbecues, and restrooms. Just past Vaca Flat is Salsipuedes Bay, a deep canyon offering a spectacular view of the sculptured pinnacles of sandstone rock towering above the lake. East of Salsipuedes Bay the lake narrows and makes a sharp S-curve.

East of the turns, the lake widens. On the south bank is McNeil Canyon, a Y-shaped canyon with a lush riparian habitat and a forest of oaks and pines. Land on the beach at the head of the left fork and walk a short distance up the canyon. During winter, a small waterfall flows over a steep wall of sandstone. Relax for a moment in the quiet solitude and listen to the gentle trickle of water flowing over the rocks.

At the east end of the lake, a delta has formed at the confluence of the Salinas River and the lake. If the lake level is high, follow the meandering stream through the swampy habitat. The environment is rich in wildlife. Egrets, herons, ducks, turtles, and frogs live in the shallow waters and thick grasses along the shoreline.

From the headwaters, follow the north shoreline of the lake back toward the west. On the right are Parola and Cold canyons, two narrow arms. During the springtime the surface of the water in these shallow arms is often covered with a thick algae bloom. Proceed through an S-curve and land at the Sapwi Boat Camp. *Sapwi* means "home of the deer" in Chumash. The camp is located on a grassy headland. The campsites are spacious and shaded with broad oaks. Pit toilets, picnic tables, and a community fire-ring are provided. The Sapwi Trail begins at the campground and connects with the Blinn Ranch Trail, which extends the entire length of the lake. The trail offers spectacular views of the lake and the surrounding mountains. Whenever hiking in remote areas watch out for snakes, ticks, and poison oak. Though seldom seen, mountain lions inhabit the mountains and canyons surrounding the lake. These beautiful creatures should be treated with respect and be given plenty of space to go about their business. Report any sighting to the park ranger.

From the Sapwi Boat Camp continue along the north shore. Jackass Canyon is one of the deeper canyons on the lake, with two narrow arms penetrating outcrops of sandstone. Vegetation is mostly chaparral and sage. Next is White Oak Bay, a wide, shallow bay surrounded by oaks and grasslands. Across the lake is the White Oak Flat launch ramp and picnic area.

At the west end of the lake, separated from the main body of the lake by a narrow arm of land, is Salinas Bay. This wide bay is surrounded by rolling hills

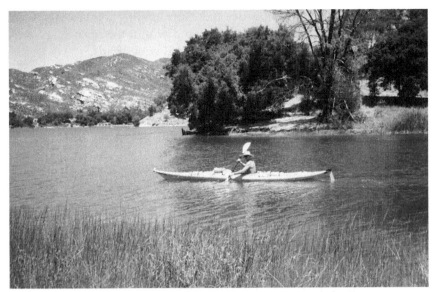

Cove adjacent to the launch site at White Oak Flat, Santa Margarita Lake

vegetated with oaks, pines and grasslands. In a narrow channel at the west end of the bay is the Salinas Dam. Passage into the channel is prohibited.

From Salinas Bay return to the launch site, following the south shore. On the broad point of land separating Murphy's Bay and Blinn Bay are the marina, campgrounds, and park headquarters. Restrooms, a store, picnic facilities, and a launch ramp are available. White Oak Flat is a short distance east of the marina.

Landing

Land at the launch ramp or on the beach at White Oak Flat.

What to do afterward

Twenty five miles of trails surround Santa Margarita Lake. Other recreational activities include fishing and sailing. Swimming is not permitted in the lake; however, there is a swimming pool, which is open from Memorial Day through September.

Alternate tour: LR3

For more information

Santa Margarita Lake Regional Park (805) 438-5485

TOUR LR3   LOPEZ LAKE, SAN LUIS OBISPO COUNTY

Tour Details	
Skill level:	Beginner
Trip length:	14.3 miles; round-trip; five to six hours
Chart/map:	Maps are available at the park entrance; USGS *Tar Springs Ridge* 7.5 min series

Summary

During spring the lake is usually full and the wildflowers are in bloom at this picturesque lake nestled in the rugged Santa Lucia Mountains of San Luis Obispo County. Lopez Lake is open daily. Swimming is permitted.

How to get there

To reach Lopez Lake Recreational Area exit Highway 101 at Grand Avenue in Arroyo Grande. Go east approximately one mile, through the city of Arroyo Grande, to Lopez Drive. Go right (east) on Lopez Drive about 10 miles to the Lopez Lake Recreational Area. Park in the parking lot at Mallard Cove. Restrooms, picnic facilities, phones, a store, and a launch ramp are provided. Fee.

Camping

Tent and RV campsites are provided at Lopez Lake Recreational Area. For reservations call (805) 489-8019.

Hazards

Hot weather, strong gusty winds, boat traffic, submerged rocks and snags, rattlesnakes, ticks, and poison oak are all possible hazards. The surface area of the lake fluctuates with varying water level. Be sure to call ahead for current lake level. This tour describes conditions at a relatively high water level.

Public access

The shoreline of the lake is within the Lopez Lake Recreational Area and is accessible to the public.

Kayak surfing

None

Launching

Launch from the sand beach or the launch ramp at Mallard Cove. Be courteous to other boaters by moving quickly away from the ramp after launching.

Tour description

Lopez Lake is long and narrow and surrounded by steep, rugged mountains. The area is mostly undeveloped with the exception of the recreational facilities (campgrounds and marina) at the southeast corner end of the lake. The lake's primary water sources are Arroyo Grande Creek, Lopez Creek, and Wittenberg Creek.

From Mallard Cove, head north toward the headwaters of Wittenberg Arm. On the right are group campgrounds and an equestrian staging area. Before the Lopez Dam was constructed this scenic valley was settled by the Wittenberg family. According to one account, the last grizzly bear killed in San Luis Obispo County was shot by by Newt Wittenberg as he stood on his front porch.

As you approach the upper reaches of Wittenberg Arm, the channel narrows and a delta has formed where the silt-laden stream joins the lake. Cattails and tule, shaded by the towering sycamores, flourish along the shoreline, and a variety of wildlife including beavers, egrets, herons, ducks, geese, turtles, and frogs can be seen in the shallow waters. French Camp, a Boy Scout camp, is located at the inlet of Wittenberg Creek.

From French Camp return south following the shoreline counterclockwise. Cormorants and grebes perch high on the barren limbs of a dead sycamore, and a group of white pelicans glide effortlessly across the smooth water. At Miller's Cove is a floating dock and the trailhead for the Two Waters Trail, a pathway connecting Wittenberg Arm to Lopez Arm. The trail offers spectacular vistas of the lake and mountains.

From Wittenberg Arm, enter the Arroyo Grande Arm and follow the northern shoreline to Lopez Arm. The earliest inhabitants of Lopez Canyon were the Chumash Indians. Their village stretched along the banks of Lopez Creek, now deep below the waters of the lake. The Chumash hunted, fished, and gathered acorns, which they ground into meal. The meal was soaked in brine water to leach out the bitter tannins, then boiled and eaten as mush or prepared into flatbread. With the coming of the missionaries in the late 1700s, the Chumash villages were abandoned, and the Franciscan Fathers from the Mission San Luis Obispo grew wheat in the secluded canyon. In 1901 the Santa Manuela schoolhouse was built at the site of what is now Lopez Dam. The old schoolhouse is presently preserved at the park marina.

The walls of Lopez Canyon are steep and covered with a wide variety of plant communities including oak woodland, grassland, chaparral, and coastal sage scrub. Flora unique to both southern and northern California are found

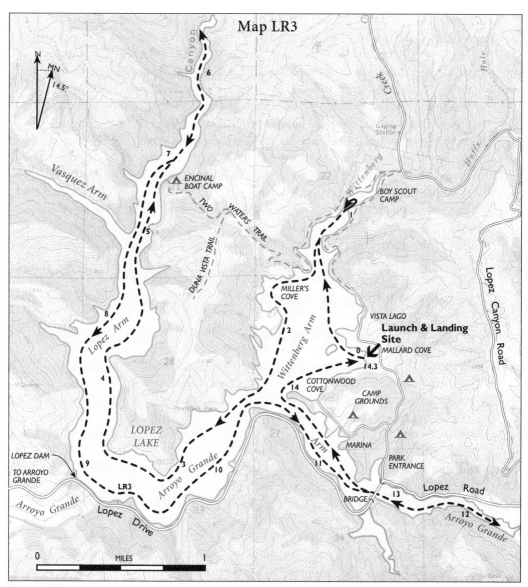

Tour LR3: Lopez Lake, San Luis Obispo County

in the area. Beginning in late February lupine, shooting star, canyon sunflower, and indian paintbrush bloom on the grassy hillsides. Wildlife in the area include deer, raccoons, squirrels, skunks, coyotes, and snakes. Black bears, bobcats, and mountain lions are seen on rare occasions.

About two thirds of the way up the Lopez Arm (on the eastern shore) is a primitive campground for use by boaters and hikers, with pit toilets and a floating dock. At the confluence of Lopez Creek and the lake is a riparian habitat similar to the one in Wittenberg Arm.

Return along the western shoreline of the arm. On the right is Vasquez Arm, a deep, narrow waterway named after Antonio Vasquez, who homesteaded 120 acres of land in the canyon in 1904. Several large scars on the ridge above Vasquez Canyon are all that remain of oil exploration activities that took place in the 1930s and again in the 1960s. Lopez Dam was completed in 1969 at a cost of 18 million dollars. The reservoir, which was supposed to take five to ten years to fill, spilled just five months after completion due to an unusually wet winter. Today the reservoir serves as a water supply for parts of San Luis Obispo County.

From the dam, follow the southern shoreline of the Arroyo Grande Arm toward the marina. Interesting exposures of sedimentary rocks of the Monterey Formation can be seen in the steep road cuts along Lopez Drive. The sediments, which were deposited on the seafloor of a warm, shallow sea some 26 million years ago, have been folded, faulted, uplifted, and eroded, forming the landscape we see today. Fossilized scallops, sand dollars, and oysters can be found along the shoreline.

Pass Wittenberg Arm and head into the eastern extension of the Arroyo Grande Arm. A store and restrooms are available at the Marina. Continue southeast past the Lopez Drive bridge and into the riparian wetlands of the Arroyo Grande Arm. During low lake levels it may not be possible to proceed beyond the Lopez Drive bridge.

Return to Wittenberg Arm and follow the south shoreline back to Mallard Cove.

Landing
Land at either the launch ramp or on the beach at Mallard Cove.

What to do afterward
There are several maintained hiking trails in the Lopez Lake Recreational Area. Other recreational activities include fishing, sailing, biking, wind surfing, water skiing, and a water slide.

Alternate tour: LR2

For more information
Lopez Lake Recreational Area (805) 489-2095

TOUR LR4 MAMMOTH POOL RESERVOIR, FRESNO/MADERA COUNTIES

Tour Details

Skill level:	Beginner
Trip length/type:	12.5 miles; round-trip; four to five hours
Chart/map:	Maps are available at Wagner's Store; USGS *Mammoth Pool Dam* 7.5 min series

Summary

Towering, forested peaks surround this secluded reservoir on the west slope of the Sierra Nevada. During winter, the road to Mammoth Pool is closed. The reservoir is also closed to the public from May 1 to June 16 to allow migrating deer to swim across the lake. Swimming is permitted. Speed limits are controlled.

How to get there

To reach Mammoth Pool Reservoir, exit Highway 41 approximately 20 miles north of Fresno at North Fork Road (O'Neals). Go east to the town of

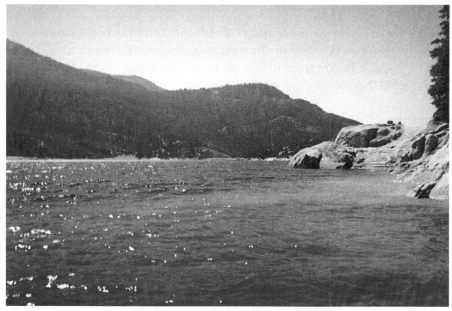

Slabs of granite rock ascend from the greenish-blue water at Mammoth Pool Reservoir

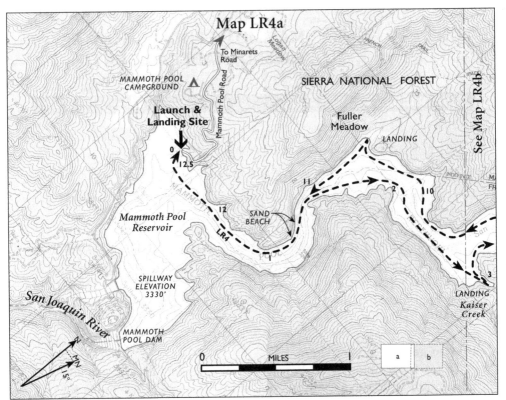

Tour LR4: Mammoth Pool Reservoir, Fresno/Madera Counties

North Fork. Turn right on Minarets Road and continue east (about 25-30 miles) to Mammoth Pool Road. Turn right on Mammoth Pool Road and proceed to the lake. Parking, restrooms, phones, a store, gas, and a launch ramp are available. No fee.

Camping

Seven Forest Service campgrounds and one privately owned campground (Wagner's Mammoth Pool Resort) are located within 13 miles of Mammoth Pool Reservoir. For information about Forest Service camping, call (209) 323-3839. For information about Wagner's call (209) 841-3736. China Bar is a primitive campground accessible by boat only.

Hazards

Hot summer weather, strong gusty winds, cold water and submerged rocks and snags are all possible hazards. The surface area of the lake fluctuates with the water level. Be sure to call ahead for current lake levels. This tour describes conditions at a relatively high water level. Fire danger at Mammoth Pool is

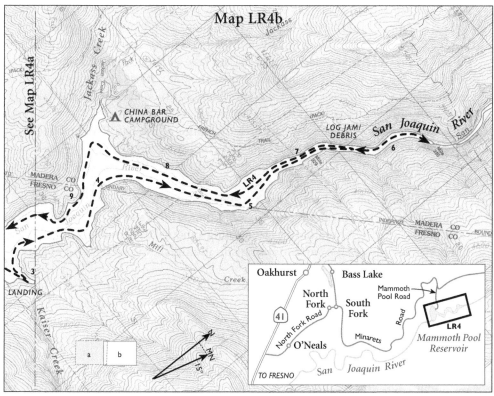

Tour LR4 (continued)

extreme during the summer. Campfire permits are required outside of developed campgrounds.

Public access
Most of the lake shoreline is within Sierra National Forest and is accessible to the public.

Kayak surfing
None

Launching
Launch from the beach or the launch ramp at the end of Mammoth Pool Road.

Tour description
Mammoth Pool Reservoir is about 90 miles northeast of Fresno on the west slope of the southern Sierra Nevada. The lake is formed behind a dam on the

San Joaquin River at an elevation of 3300 feet. It was named after a (former) large natural pool in the river just above the dam. The dam has a maximum storage capacity of 120,000 acre feet and is operated by Southern California Edison to produce hydroelectric power. The lake is about five and one-half miles long and up to one-half mile wide near the dam. It has a sinuous shape and few major tributaries except the San Joaquin River that enters the lake from the northeast; the dam is to the southwest.

From the launch ramp head east into the gorge of the San Joaquin River. Along the shoreline, huge, rounded slabs of granite ascend from the greenish-blue water. The warm, still air and deep-blue sky provide the picture-perfect setting.

At about one mile the lake makes a 90-degree turn to the north. On the left bank is a sandy beach offering an easy landing. The water is exceptionally clear and a good temperature for swimming (about 70 degrees during the summer). The rays of the early morning sun illuminate the white sand at the bottom of the lake.

About one mile ahead the lake makes another 90-degree turn. On the left bank is Fuller Meadow, a beautiful, green, mountain meadow surrounded by towering ponderosa pine, and incense cedars. A careful observer may catch a glimpse of California mule deer grazing in the lush meadow. On the right shoreline is a prominent outcropping of granite. East of Fuller Meadow is Kaiser Creek, a tributary entering the lake from the southeast. During the spring, the roar of the cascading water can be heard nearly a half-mile away. Landing is possible on the sandy beach adjoining the creek. This remote location is forested with a variety of pines intermingled with live and black oak.

At Kaiser Creek the lake once again veers north. Jackass Creek and the China Bar primitive boat camp are on the north shore about one mile north of Kaiser Creek. From China Bar the lake follows a relatively narrow, northeast trending canyon. The Fuller Buttes, two rounded domes of granite towering high above the canyon, reflect perfectly in the mirror-smooth water. The canyon continues to narrow until the lake is only a couple of hundred feet wide. The granite walls are nearly vertical and landing spots are limited. Pick your way through the logjam of floating wood that obstructs the narrow channel. The water is very clear and cold, and a slight turbulence can be detected. Soon the roar of rushing water echoes off the canyon walls. Around the next bend is the mighty San Joaquin River spilling into the lake over the piles of rounded granite boulders. To view the river in its natural setting (above the high-water level of the lake), climb to the top of the rock pile that forms the end of lake. The smooth, wet rocks are very slippery so be careful.

Return from the headwaters to the launch site.

Landing
Land at the launch ramp or the adjoining beach.

What to do afterward

Mammoth Pool reservoir is noted for its hiking, fishing, and boating. Rainbow, eastern brook, and brown trout are landed during the fishing season, which extends from mid-April to late fall when the road is closed. The French Trail, built by John S. French in 1880 to service mines in the Mammoth Mountain area, parallels the northwest shoreline. The trail begins at Ross' Ranch and ends just south of the Devils Postpile near Mammoth Lakes.

Alternate tour: LR1

For more information

US Forest Service, Sierra National Forest, Minarets Ranger District
(209) 877-2218

TOUR LR5 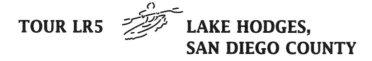 LAKE HODGES, SAN DIEGO COUNTY

Tour Details	
Skill level:	Beginner
Trip length/type:	14.0 miles; round-trip; five to six hours
Chart/map:	Maps are available at the lake concession; USGS *Escondido* 7.5 min series

Summary

Located only minutes from north San Diego County's coastal communities, Lake Hodges is a favorite spot for local kayakers. Lake Hodges is open Wednesday, Saturday, and Sunday from sunrise to sunset. Call to verify the current schedule. Swimming is not permitted.

How to get there

To reach Lake Hodges, exit Interstate 15 at Via Rancho Parkway near Escondido and proceed west to Lake Drive. Go left on Lake Drive to the lake entrance on the left. Park in the lot adjacent to the concession stand. Restrooms, picnic facilities, a snack bar, launch ramp, and phones are available. Fee.

Camping

Overnight camping is not available at Lake Hodges.

Hazards

Hot weather, strong, gusty winds, boat traffic, submerged rocks, and snags, rattlesnakes, ticks, and poison oak are all possible hazards. The surface area of the lake fluctuates with varying water level. Be sure to call ahead for current lake level. This tour describes conditions at a relatively high water level.

Public access

Most of the shoreline is accessible to the public.

Kayak surfing

None

Launching

Launch from either of the two launch ramps or from the beach adjacent to the ramp. Be courteous to other boaters by moving quickly away from the ramp after launching.

Tour description

From the launch site, proceed northwest. The western arm of the lake is in a long, narrow valley. Follow the western shoreline south toward the dam. Vegetation along the shore consists of lush riparian marshland, with open

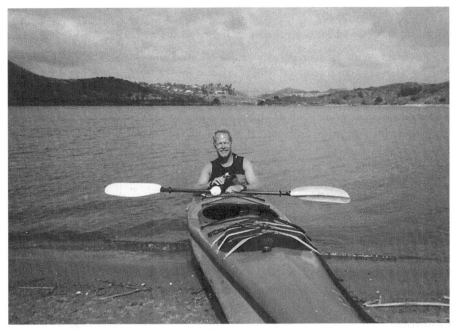

Sheltered rest stop at Bernardo Bay, Lake Hodges, San Diego County

grassland, scrub oak, and chaparral on the hillside above. Lake Drive is developed with residences and a few commercial establishments. Fishing is popular, and so are the bike path and and hiking trail that parallel the shoreline. Strong afternoon winds, make the western arm of the lake a favorite spot for wind surfers.

Cross the lake at the dam and return along the undeveloped, eastern shoreline. Walls of solid granite rise steeply from the water's edge. Ferns, wildflowers, and scrub oak cling to the shaded slopes and spring-fed water (during the spring) trickles from the granite ledges.

Continue around the narrow peninsula of land separating the west and east arms of the lake. Just past the marina is the *SS Relief*, a floating restroom. Approximately one-half mile east of the marina, the lake narrows. Power boats are required to reduce speed to less than ten miles per hour to minimize wake. Paddle close to the shoreline and watch for boat traffic when paddling through the narrows. About one and one-half miles southeast of the launch ramp is Bernardo Bay. The bay is somewhat sheltered from the wind and there are several good landing sites along the southwest shore. A scenic hiking trail meanders through the trees and grasslands. During spring the wildflowers are abundant. Watch out for snakes and poison oak.

At the head of Bernardo Bay a narrow channel winds through the shallow marshland. Follow the channel as far as you can go. The water is still and the vegetation lush and green. Snowy egrets nest in the marsh grass. Close your eyes and enjoy the silence.

From Bernardo Bay continue east, following the main channel of the lake. Ahead is the Interstate 15 overpass. The roar of traffic can be heard from over a mile away. If you have never paddled beneath a freeway, give it a try. To the east of Interstate 15 the water is very shallow and often impassable when the water level in the lake is low.

Return beneath the freeway and follow the north shoreline of the lake back toward the launch site. During the afternoon you may encounter a headwind. Follow the shoreline closely to minimize the chop.

Landing

Land at the launch ramp or on the beach adjacent to the ramp.

What to do afterward

Lake Hodges offers fifteen miles of scenic hiking and biking trails, fishing, and wind surfing.

Alternate tour: LR6

For more information

San Diego City Lakes Information (619) 465-3474

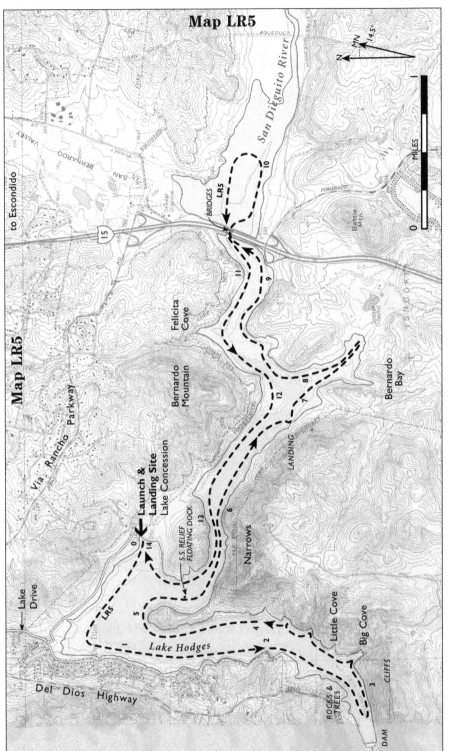

Map LR5

Tour LR5: Lake Hodges, San Diego County

TOUR LR6   LAKE MORENA, SAN DIEGO COUNTY

Tour Details

Skill level:	Beginner
Trip length/type:	8.5 miles; round-trip; three to four hours
Chart/map:	Maps are available at the ranger headquarters; USGS Morena Reservoir 7.5 min series

Summary

3,250 acres of spectacular wilderness parkland surround Lake Morena, the highest and most remote of San Diego's reservoirs. The lake is open daily. Jet skis, water skiing, and swimming are not permitted.

How to get there

To reach Lake Morena from the San Diego area, exit Interstate 8 approximately 31 miles of east of El Cajon at Buckman Springs Road (Highway S1). Proceed south on Buckman Springs road to Oak Drive and go right to Lake Morena Drive. Go right on Lake Morena Drive and follow the signs to Lake Morena Regional Park. Park in the lot adjacent to the launch ramp. Restrooms, picnic facilities, and telephones are available. Fee.

Camping

Tent and RV campsites are available at Lake Morena Regional Park. For camping reservations, call (619) 565-3600.

Hazards

Hot weather, strong gusty winds, boat traffic, submerged rocks and snags, rattlesnakes, ticks, and poison oak are all possible hazards. The surface area of the lake fluctuates with varying water level. Be sure to call ahead for current lake level. This tour describes conditions at a relatively high water level.

Public access

The shoreline of the lake is within Lake Morena Regional Park and is accessible to the public.

Kayak surfing

None

Launching

Launch from the beach or from the public launch ramp at Lake Morena Regional Park. A floating dock is available for loading gear. Be courteous to other boaters by moving quickly away from the ramp after launching.

Tour description

From the boat launch, proceed west toward the dam. It's best to begin your trip in the morning, before the westerly wind begins to blow. If you get a late start, this leg of the trip could be a long, difficult paddle, directly into the wind.

The Lake Morena Dam is constructed across a narrow gap in the high granite ridge that parallels the western shoreline of the lake. Bald eagles can be seen soaring high above the ridge in the vicinity of the dam. Several hiking trails follow the south shoreline from the launch site to the dam. This arm of the lake is the deepest and is suitable for boating even at a low water level. Because the surrounding mountains are mostly solid granite, there is little sediment in the runoff and the water visibility is usually good.

From the dam, head back toward the launch site along the north shore. On the left is a wide embayment with a riparian habitat at the headwaters. Cottonwood trees flourish in the moist environment. When you are opposite the launch ramp, head north following the western shoreline of the Morena Arm. A variety of birds roost on the rocks and small islands. Vegetation surrounding Lake Morena displays characteristics of desert, coastal, and mountain habitats; chaparral and scrub oak at higher elevations, and grasslands and riparian communities along the shoreline. Prior to the 1800s, the area was inhabited by the Kumeyaay Indians. Smooth, round bowls used for grinding acorns into meal can still be seen in the hard granite rock. Because the area is remote, rare predators such as mountain lions and bobcats are occasionally observed. More common forms of wildlife seen in the park include mule deer, coyotes, raccoons, striped and spotted skunks, rattlesnakes, and brush rabbits. Trout fishing is good in winter and the bass begin biting in spring.

Continue following the shoreline clockwise around Goat Island. On the peninsula to the east is the North Shore primitive campground. A strong westerly wind can generate choppy conditions along the west side of the peninsula. Round the peninsula and head into Cottonwood Arm. The east shore of the peninsula is sheltered from the westerly wind and several sandy coves offer suitable landing.

Cottonwood Creek is one of the main tributaries of the lake. The creek flows from a broad valley vegetated with grasslands, oaks, and cottonwood trees. At the inlet of the creek is a delta with a riparian habitat supporting a variety of wildlife including egrets, herons, ducks, turtles, and frogs.

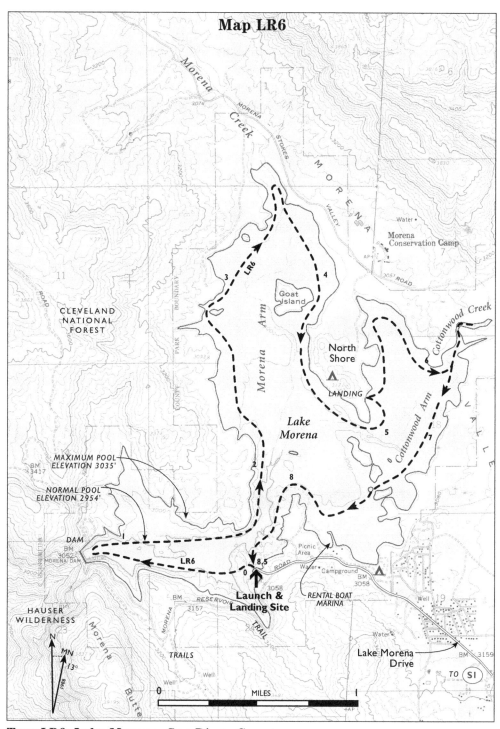

Tour LR6: Lake Morena, San Diego County

From Cottonwood Creek head southeast along the east shoreline of Cottonwood Arm. The water is shallow and the shoreline is a marshland with several low, grassy islands. During low water, much of this part of the lake is inaccessible. A headwind may be encountered when returning to the launch site from Cottonwood Arm. When possible, paddle in the lee of the headlands to avoid the chop. On the left is the Lake Morena campground and the rental-boat marina. Private boats are not permitted to land at the rental-boat dock. Follow the shoreline around the rocky headland to the launch ramp.

Landing
Land at the boat ramp or on the beach adjacent to the ramp.

What to do afterward
Lake Morena Regional Park offers numerous nature trails including the Pacific Crest Trail, which extends all the way from Mexico to Canada. For a glimpse of the past, visit the historic San Diego Railroad Museum and the century-old Gaskill Stone Store Museum in the nearby community of Campo.

Alternate tour: LR5

For more information
San Diego County Department of Parks and Recreation (619) 694-3049

TOUR LR7 TOPOCK GORGE, COLORADO RIVER, SAN BERNARDINO COUNTY

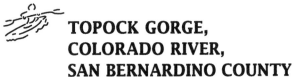

Tour Details	
Skill level:	Beginner
Trip length/type:	16.6 miles; one-way; five to six hours
Chart/map:	Maps are available at the park entrance; USGS *Topock* and *Castle Rock* 7.5 min series

Summary
This journey through the steep, red-rock canyon of the Havasu National Wildlife Refuge, is in one of the most beautiful sections of the Colorado River.

How to get there
To reach the launch site, exit Interstate 40, eleven miles southeast of Needles at Moabi Regional Park. Restrooms, picnic facilities, a launch ramp, and phones are available. Fee.

To reach the landing site, exit Interstate 40 about ten miles east of the Colorado River (in Arizona) at Highway 95. Go south to London Bridge Drive. Go right to Fathom Drive. Go right to Reef Drive. Go left to the Castle Rock Landing and park in the gravel parking area. The landing site is about 200 yards from the parking area at the end of a gravel trail. Go to the end of the trail to view the landing site so you know what to look for at the end of the trip. No facilities are available. No fee.

Camping

Tent and RV campsites are available at Moabi Regional Park. For reservations call (760) 326-3831.

Hazards

Hot weather, strong, gusty winds, cold water, strong currents, boat traffic, submerged rocks and snags, and rattlesnakes are all possible hazards. Take plenty of water to prevent dehydration. Flash flooding can occur in the side channels following a thunderstorm.

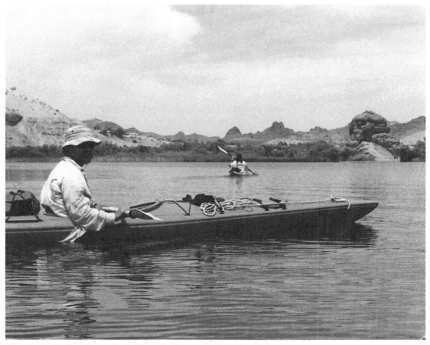

Castle Rock (landing site), Topock Gorge, Colorado River

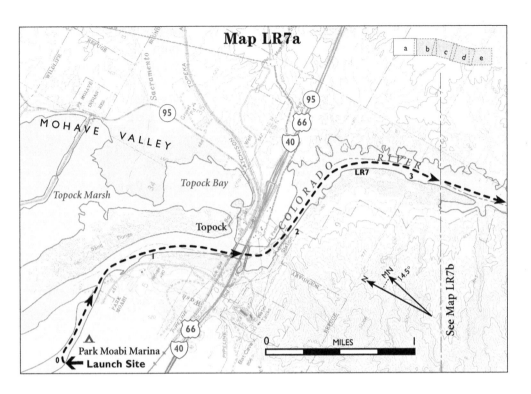

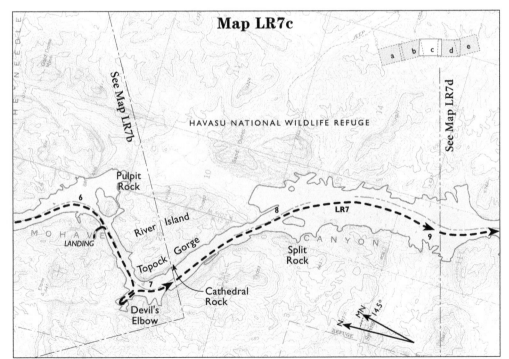

Tour LR7: Topock Gorge, Colorado River, San Bernardino County

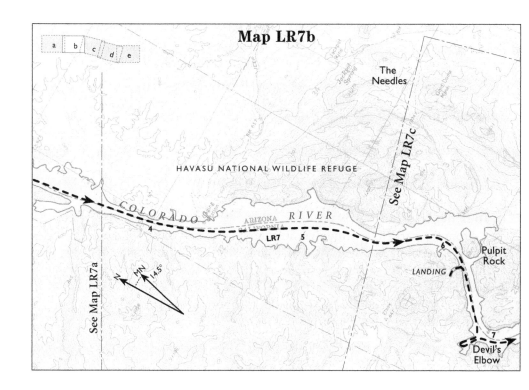

Map LR7b

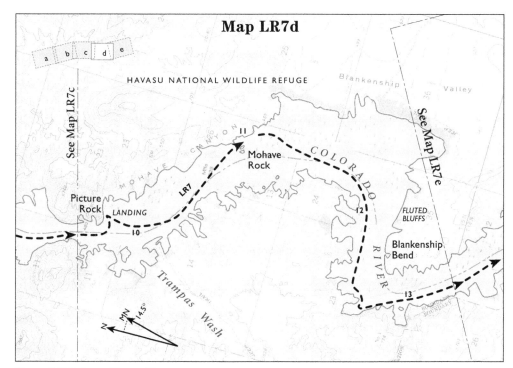

Map LR7d

Tour LR7 (continued)

Public access

Most of the shoreline is accessible to the public by boat but not by car. Some portions of the shoreline are designated as fragile riparian wildlife preserves landing is not allowed.

Kayak surfing

None

Launching

Launch from the beach at Moabi Regional Park.

Tour description

From the park, follow the river inlet about one-half mile to the main channel of the Colorado River. At about one and one-half mile you will reach Interstate 40 and the Santa Fe railroad bridges. Beneath the bridges a buoy line marks the north boundary of the Topock Gorge Unit of the Havasu National Wildlife Refuge. No water skiing, open fires, or overnight camping are permitted within the refuge.

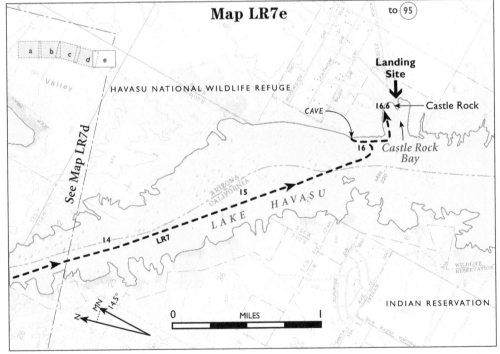

Tour LR7 (continued)

At about three miles, the surrounding terrain becomes more mountainous. High above the east shore of the river are the distinctive Needles Peaks, visible throughout the region. The turquoise water and the green vegetation hugging the river bank provide a stark contrast to the surrounding desert environment. Rare birds and wildlife inhabit the marshlands adjoining the river, and bighorn sheep can occasionally be spotted on the steep, rocky slopes.

At Pulpit Rock the river makes a sharp bend to the right. Just around the bend is a protected landing with a sand beach. A dirt path leads from the beach to a rocky point offering a spectacular vista of the gorge. Approximately one-half mile beyond Pulpit Rock is the Devil's Elbow, a sharp 90-degree turn to the left. The section of river between Pulpit Rock and Devil's Elbow is spectacular, with vertical walls of red volcanic rock ascending from the swirling turquoise water. Narrow side canyons lead to isolated coves with sandy beaches.

From Devil's Elbow, the river follows a relatively straight course south. East of the river are several large sand dunes and to the west is a wildlife preserve. Landing is prohibited in certain areas of the preserve. At about nine and three-quarter miles is Picture Rock, a prominent headland on the east shore. Indian petroglyphs carved into the face of the rock describe the lifestyle of the *Aha Makaav* (Mojave) Indians who inhabited the area for thousands of years. The protected site is referred to as *Hom Me Chomp,* which means "The rock where the river once churned to make this place inaccessible to the living."

South of Picture Rock the narrow gorge opens into a broad valley. Tributaries meander across the marshlands bordering the river. At 11 miles is Mohave Rock, an immense rock monolith on the east shore. A shallow-water inlet flows east around Mojave Rock, then returns to the main channel about one-quarter mile downstream.

Blankenship Bend is another sharp turn in the river. The sandy ridge on the east shoreline has interesting vertical erosional features called the fluted bluffs. A large still-water embayment on the west side of the river at Blankenship Bend provides a good landing site. South of Blankenship Bend, the river follows a relatively straight southward course. The river is wide and there is considerable boat traffic coming up-river from Lake Havasu. At about 15 miles you will see several homes on the hills to the east. Cross to the eastern shore and watch for the *Castle Rock* sign.

Follow the inlet marked *Castle Rock* for about one-quarter mile to a vertical bluff. Head north along the narrow channel at the foot of the bluff for about one-quarter mile. On the right is a cave, passable in a kayak. After exploring the cave, follow the channel back to the south, past where you first reached the vertical bluff. A side channel heading east is identified by a row of buoys. The channel leads to a large bay. Across the bay is a low, dark, rock outcropping known as Castle Rock.

Landing

Land on the gravel beach adjacent to Castle Rock.

What to do afterward

Topock Marsh, part of Havasu National Wildlife Refuge, consists of a network of shallow river channels, sloughs, and swamps perfect for exploring in a kayak. Several species of migratory birds have nesting rookeries in the marsh, and fishing for bass, catfish, and trout can be excellent. Historic London Bridge is in Lake Havasu City, about six miles south of Castle Rock. The City of Laughlin, 24 miles north of Needles offers riverfront gambling casinos.

Alternate tour: None

For more information

Havasu National Wildlife Refuge (619) 326-3853

Appendix 1
Central and Southern California Kayak Retailer List

Retailer	Location	Telephone
Crystal Point	Agoura Hills	(818) 707-2991
Sierra Nevada Adventures	Arnold	(209) 795-9310
Descanso Beach Ocean Sports	Avalon	(310) 510-1226
Sailboats of Bakersfield	Bakersfield	(805) 322-9178
Glen-L Marine Designs	Bellflower	(310) 630-6258
Sport Chalet	Brea	(714) 255-0132
Sport Chalet	Burbank	(818) 558-3500
California Watersports	Carlsbad	(619) 434-3089
Carlsbad Paddle Sports	Carlsbad	(760) 434-8686
Metro	Carlsbad	(619) 729-0895
Ocean Quest Kayak Center	Carlsbad	(619) 431-0895
Murray Watersports	Carpenteria	(805) 786-7245
REI	Carson	(310) 538-2429
Good Clean Fun	Cayucos	(805) 995-1993
UP Sports	Dana Point	(714) 443-5161
Southern Stars	Dana Point	(714) 489-0059
Sport Chalet	El Cajon	(619) 590-9099
Ocean Master	El Monte	(626) 582-8000
Pacific Eagle USA	El Monte	(626) 455-0033
Big 5 Sporting Goods	El Segundo	
Paddler's Supply Company	Escondido	(619) 739-8383
California Outfitters	Fresno	
Herb Bauer Sporting Goods	Fresno	(209) 435-8600
Sailing Center	Friant	(209) 822-2666
Sport Chalet	Glendora	(818) 335-3344
Aquatics Dive Locker	Goleta	(805) 964-8680
Echo Sports	Huntington Beach	(714) 960-4007
Sport Chalet	Huntington Beach	(714) 848-0988
Silverstrand Sea Sports	Imperial Beach	(619) 437-3043
Southwind Kayak Center	Irvine	(714) 261-0200
Sport Chalet	Irvine	(714) 476-9555
Mountain and River Adventure	Kernville	(800) 861-6553
Sierra South Inc.	Kernville	(760) 376-3745
Sport Chalet	La Canada	(818) 790-9800
Sports Chalet Water Sports Center	La Jolla	(619) 552-0712

What in the World	Lake Arrowhead	(909) 337-5080
Teamsports	Lawndale	(310) 371-8019
Koala Kauak	Lompoc	(805) 886-8888
Long Beach Windsurf Center	Long Beach	(562) 433-1014
Canoe Pacific	Los Angeles	(310) 397-4092
Sport Chalet	Los Angeles	(310) 657-3210
Summit Sportswear	Los Angeles	(310) 479-8892
White Water Express	Los Angeles	(310) 820-1103
Malibu Ocean Sports	Malibu	(310) 456-6302
Zuma Jay	Malibu	(310) 456-8044
Caldera Kayaks	Mammoth Lakes	(619) 935-4942
Sandy's Ski and Sport	Mammoth Lakes	(619) 934-7518
River Sea West	Manhattan Beach	(310) 372-8305
Action Watersports	Marina del Rey	(310) 827-2233
California Surf and Kayak	Marina del Rey	(310) 301-2426
Sport Chalet	Marina del Rey	(310) 821-9400
REI	Mission Viejo	(714) 348-1400
Sport Chalet	Mission Viejo	(714) 582-3363
Valley Sporting Goods	Modesto	(209) 523-5681
Sport Chalet	Montclair	(919) 946-1517
Adventures by the Sea	Monterey	(408) 372-1807
Monterey Bay Kayaks	Monterey	(408) 373-5357
Kayak Horizons	Morro Bay	(805) 772-6444
SNAC	Murphy's	(209) 532-5621
Seda Kayaks	National City	(619) 336-2444
Paddle Power	Newport Beach	(714) 675-1215
REI	Northridge	(818) 831-5555
Sport Chalet	Oxnard	(805) 485-5222
Sport Chalet	Rancho Cucamonga	(909) 987-4321
Mainstream	Redondo Beach	(310) 316-2099
The Kayak Store	Redondo Beach	(310) 318-1717
Pacific Legends	Reseda	(818) 342-3694
Adventure 16	San Diego	(619) 283-6314
Canoyon Sports Racks	San Diego	(619) 676-1950
Mission Bay Paddle Sports	San Diego	(619) 488-5599
REI	San Diego	(619) 279-4400
San Diego Sailing Center/Kayak	San Diego	(619) 488-0651
Southwest Sea Kayaks	San Diego	(619) 222-3616
Sport Chalet	San Diego	(619) 224-6777
Sport Chalet Watersports Center	San Diego	(619) 552-0712
Windsport	San Diego	(619) 488-4642
REI	San Dimas	(909) 592-2095

Pacific Marine	San Luis Obispo	(805) 544-4471
REI	Santa Ana	(714) 543-4142
Harbor Watersports Center	Santa Barbara	(805) 962-4890
Paddle Sports of Santa Barbara	Santa Barbara	(805) 899-4925
Santa Barbara Aquatics	Santa Barbara	(805) 964-8689
"Two Harbors"	Santa Catalina Island	(310) 510-0303
Sport Chalet	Santa Clara	(805) 253-3883
Adventure Sports	Santa Cruz	(408) 458-3648
Kayak Connection	Santa Cruz	(408) 479-1121
Venture Quest	Santa Cruz	(408) 427-2267
Dive West Sports	Santa Maria	(805) 925-5878
Dive Shop of Santa Maria	Santa Maria	(805) 922-0076
Watersports Safari	Shaver Lake	(209) 841-8222
Central Coast Kayaks	Shell Beach	(805) 773-3500
Sports Chalet	Torrance	(310) 316-6634
Crescenta Valley Canoe	Tujunga	(818) 957-3922
Sport Chalet	Valencia	(805) 253-3883
Real Cheap Sports	Ventura	(805) 648-3803
Trip Canoes and Kayaks	Ventura	(805) 643-8856
Sport Chalet	West Hills	(818) 710-0999
Xstreamline Sports	Wilmington	(310) 518-1972
Sports Ltd.	Woodland Hills	(818) 225-7669

Appendix 2
Selected References

Badaracco, Robert, *Lopez Guide*. San Luis Obispo, CA: County of San Luis Obispo 1984

Bunnell, David, *Sea Caves of Santa Cruz Island*. Santa Barbara, CA: McNally & Loftin, Publishers. 1991.

Bunnell, David, *Sea Caves of Anacapa Island*. Santa Barbara, CA: McNally & Loftin, Publishers. 1993.

Burch, David, *Fundamentals of Kayak Navigation*. The Globe Pequot Press. 1987

California Coastal Commission. *California Coastal Access Guide*. Berkeley, CA: University of California Press. 1997.

California Coastal Commission. *California Coastal Resource Guide*. Berkeley, CA: University of California Press. 1987

Department of Boating and Waterways, *ABCs of the California Boating Law*. Sacramento, CA.

Dirksen, & McKinney, *Colorado River Recreation*. Aptos, CA: Recreation Sales Publishing. 1995.

Dirksen, D.J., *Recreation Lakes of California*. Aptos, CA: Recreation Sales Publishing. 1996.

Fagan, Brian, *Cruising Guide to Southern California's Offshore Islands*. Santa Barbara, CA: Caractacus Corporation. 1993.

Griggs & Savoy, *Living With the California Coast*. Durham, NC: Duke University Press. 1985.

Miller, Bruce, *Chumash: A Picture of Their World*. Los Osos, CA: Sand River Press. 1988

Norris & Webb, *Geology of California*, New York, NY: John Wiley and Sons. 1990.

Santa Barbara Museum of Natural History, *California's Chumash Indians*, San Luis Obispo, CA: EZ Nature Books. 1988.

Seidman, David, T*he Essential Sea Kayaker*. Camden, ME: Ragged Mountain Press. 1992

Sharp, Robert, *Field Guide to Southern California*. Dubuque, IA: Wm. C. Brown Company Publishers. 1994.

Shepard, Francis, *The Earth Beneath the Sea*. Atheneum, NY: Atheneum. 1973.

Snyderman, Marty, *California Marine Life*. Port Hueneme, CA: Marcor Publishing. 1997.

Tway, Linda, *Tidepools of Southern California*. Santa Barbara, CA: Capra Press. 1991.

Walker, Doris,*Adventurer's Guide to Dana Point*. Dana Point, CA: To the Point Press. 1992

Winlund, Ed, *Chart Guide, California*. Anaheim, CA: ChartGuide Ltd. 1990.

Wyatt, Mikek, *The Basic Essentials of Sea Kayaking*. Merrillville, IN: ICS Books. 1990.

Index

About the Author

Rob Mohle's life has evolved around the water. His first nautical experiences began at a young age when his family moved to Norway and they sailed the fiords. In 1960, his family returned to California, and spent many summers on a boat at Catalina Island. In 1961 he got his first surfboard and during the next 15 years surfed the beaches of central and southern California. In 1976 he moved to San Luis Obispo County where he lives today and works as a professional geologist. Rob has two sons who continue the family's seafaring tradition.

Rob has been kayaking for over 10 years and has explored most of the coastline between Big Sur and San Diego. His love for the outdoors has led him to paddle extensively, and write numerous articles on adventure kayaking.

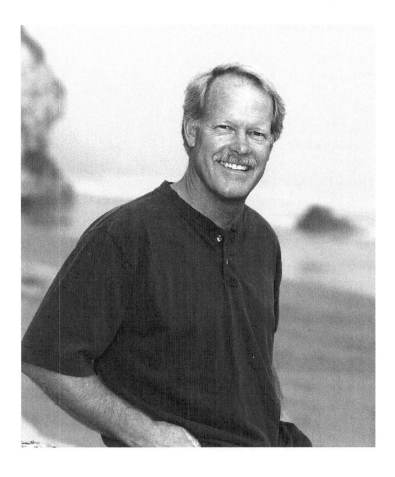

Read This!

I would appreciate hearing from readers who have spotted errors or who have suggestions or updated information. Please write to me in care of Wilderness Press.

The material in this book has been carefully prepared from many sources including, but not limited to, personal visits by the author, publications, and other information deemed reliable for the purpose of providing objective information which can be used by the reader to intelligently and safely pursue kayaking adventures along California's scenic waterways. Although every effort has been made to assure completeness and accuracy, no guidebook can alert you to every possible hazard or anticipate the abilities or limitations of every reader. Shorelines, river channels, and weather and sea conditions constantly change. The capabilities of you, your party, and your kayak cannot be predicted by the author or the publisher. The descriptions are not representations that every trip is safe for you or your party. If you decide to take one of these trips, read the entire trip description carefully before beginning the trip. The information should be considered advisory in nature and never a substitute for sound judgment and qualified instruction. You assume all risks and full responsibility for your own safety. The author and publisher disclaim any and all liability for loss or risk, to persons or to property or both, which might occur, either directly or indirectly, from any person's use of or interpretation of any information contained in this book.

Grab your paddle and put in with more guides from our *Adventure Kayaking* series...

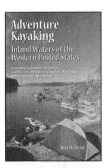

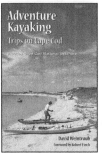

Adventure Kayaking: Inland Waters of the Western United States

Don Skillman

Discover some of the premier paddling spots on the rivers and lakes of California, Arizona, Oregon, Nevada, Utah, and Washington with 13 carefully selected trips.

Adventure Kayaking: Trips on Cape Cod and Martha's Vineyard

David Weintraub

Features 25 exciting trips covering the entire Cape from Falmouth to Provincetown, including renowned Cape Cod National Seashore, and now Martha's Vineyard.

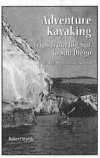

Adventure Kayaking: Trips from the Russian River to Monterey

Michael Jeneid

Explore 150 miles of beautiful lagoons, bays, and esteros of the Central California coastline from the Russian River to Monterey with this book's 24 day trips for kayak.

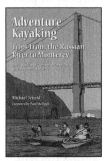

Adventure Kayaking: Trips from Big Sur to San Diego

Robert Mohle

This book has over 50 trips along the Southern California coastline. Paddle along the magnificent coast of Big Sur, among the scenic Channel Islands, and past the sparkling beaches of northern San Diego county.

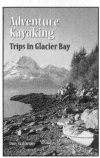

Adventure Kayaking: Trips in Glacier Bay

Don Skillman

Enjoy the deep blue glacial waters of Southeast Alaska by paddle! This book covers over 300 miles of trips in and around Glacier Bay and Glacier Bay National Park.

For more information on these and other **Wilderness Press** titles, contact us at **(800) 443-7227** or visit our website at **wildernesspress.com**